PSYCHOPATHY - NEW UPDATES ON AN OLD PHENOMENON

Edited by **Federico Durbano**

Psychopathy - New Updates on an Old Phenomenon
http://dx.doi.org/10.5772/65519
Edited by Federico Durbano

Contributors

Liane Leedom, Mehmet Hakan Turkcapar, Kadir Ozdel, Emre Sargin, Margarida Simões, Rui Abrunhosa Gonçalves, Merve Cikili, Liliana Lorettu, Giancarlo Nivoli, Alessandra M. Nivoli, Floriana Irtelli, Enrico Vincenti, Sevgi Guney, Roxana Sipos, Elena Predescu

Published by InTech

Janeza Trdine 9, 51000 Rijeka, Croatia

Publishing Process Manager Nina Kalinic
Technical Editor SPi Global
Cover InTech Design team

First published December, 2017
Printed in Croatia
Legal deposit, Croatia: National and University Library in Zagreb

Additional hard copies can be obtained from orders@intechopen.com

Psychopathy - New Updates on an Old Phenomenon, Edited by Federico Durbano
p. cm.
Print ISBN 978-953-51-3693-4
Online ISBN 978-953-51-3694-1

Meet the editor

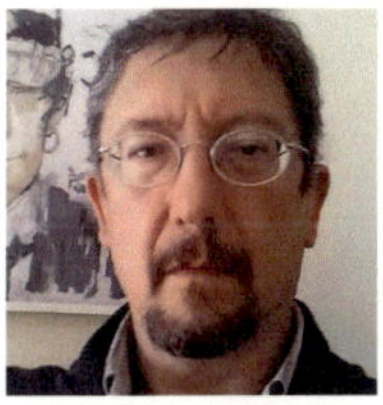

Dr. Federico Durbano was born in Genoa, Italy, in 1963, and he is living near Milan, where he received a degree in Medicine and specialized in Psychiatry. He had different work experiences in some hospitals (Milan "Ospedale Maggiore Policlinico," Treviglio, Melegnano, Fatebenefratelli), where he has achieved significant career milestones, and now he is the director of Psychiatric Unit in Melzo Hospital—ASST Melegnano e della Martesana—and vice director of Mental Health and Substance Dependence Department in the same ASST. He had teaching assignments from the University of Milan (Nursing School) and University of Castellanza (Master in Criminology). He also attended more than 70 local and national congress and courses as invited speaker, and he published more than 160 papers in national and international journals and books. He also works as technical advisor to the court in the field of forensic psychiatry.

Contents

Preface IX

Chapter 1 **From Moral Insanity to Psychopathy 1**
Liliana Lorettu, Alessandra M. Nivoli and Giancarlo Nivoli

Chapter 2 **Development of Psychopathy from Childhood 21**
Merve Cikili Uytun

Chapter 3 **The Problem of Adolescent Psychopathy: The Downward Extension of Adult Psychopathy 57**
Margarida Simões and Rui Abrunhosa Gonçalves

Chapter 4 **The Relationship between Emotional Distress and Cognitive Coping Strategies in Adolescents with Conduct Disorder (CD) 77**
Roxana Şipoş and Elena Predescu

Chapter 5 **Cognitive-Behavioral Theory and Treatment of Antisocial Personality Disorder 99**
Ahmet Emre Sargın, Kadir Özdel and Mehmet Hakan Türkçapar

Chapter 6 **Psychopathy: A Behavioral Systems Approach 117**
Liane J. Leedom

Chapter 7 **The Impact of Psychopathy on the Family 139**
Liane J. Leedom

Chapter 8 **Psychopathy: The Reflection of Severe Psychosocial Dysfunction 169**
Sevgi Güney

Chapter 9 **Successful Psychopaths: A Contemporary Phenomenon 185**
Floriana Irtelli and Enrico Vincenti

Preface

Psychopathy is considered a serious personality disorder with profound negative effects on individuals and society. The incidence of psychopathy, with significant differences according to different diagnostic criteria and population of study, varies between 0.6 and 4%, with males more represented than females. Brain imaging studies of psychopathic individuals are increasingly showing smaller and less active amygdala and specific areas in the prefrontal cortex. Other physiological derangements in psychopathy include alterations and dysregulation in neurotransmitter homeostasis (specifically dopamine and serotonin), altered endocrine responses (in particular testosterone and cortisol), and specific alterations in autonomic responses to emotional stimuli and stressors. There is also some emerging evidence of phenotypic variants in psychopathy (i.e., successful and unsuccessful types) [1]. The brain dysfunctions can be summarized as follows: lowered activity in affect-processing brain areas to emotional/salient stimuli; heightened activity in brain areas associated with reward processing and cognitive control in tasks involving moral processing, decision making, and reward; and other atypical activities in brain areas involved in social behavior [2-3]; they also showed dysfunctions in emotional regulation [4].

Hare [5], following on the seminal work of Cleckley [6], has maintained that psychopathy includes two dimensions, one involving personality development (psychological dimension) and one involving antisocial aspects (behavioral dimension). On these bases, Hare developed the most widely used diagnostic tool, the PCL (now in its R version). The tool is not perfect, however, due to the population from which it originated and to some critical diagnostic issues regarding psychopathy.

The common factor analysis of PCL-R, applied with multiple decision rules and replications, confirmed the hypnotized two-factor structure of psychopathic structure: core psychopathic personality traits (lack of remorse, shallow affect, and conning/manipulative) and antisocial lifestyle (poor behavioral controls, impulsivity, and lack of realistic long-term plans) [7-9]. The expression of the core psychopathic personality feature may be applicable across diverse morbidity and social strata, where the expression of antisocial behaviors may take different forms in different populations.

The PCL-R, however, was developed in prison and forensic psychiatry samples, and this could be a limit in its diagnostic/prognostic value. What about other populations where aspects of behavioral developments are quite different from the original populations on which the instrument was developed? Core features as need for stimulation, poor behavior controls, and irresponsibility frequently emerge in diverse groups of psychopathic individuals, but a critical issue is that it is not clear if behavioral components as parasitic lifestyle, juvenile delinquency, or lack of realistic goals would apply in the same way to all psychopathic individuals. Antisocial behaviors associated with psychopathy may take, in fact, many forms, depending on the cultural, social, or psychiatric background of the individual (e.g., the white-collar psychopath in contrast to a classical criminal subject). Although there is agreement that psychopathic personality components such as conning, manipulativeness, lack of empathy, or lack of guilt could be found in a white-collar psychopathic individual, the antisocial behaviors composing the second factor may not apply in equal degree.

Other important issues refer to the biological/social basis of antisocial behavior. It is known that psychopaths have amygdala dysfunctions, they have significant problems in aversive learning, and they do not have "normal" fear reactions and so on [10]. But how much is nature and how much is nurture? The issue has also a significant forensic pitfall: what about the freedom of choice? If all is due to nature, the individual can do nothing to react to impulse; on the contrary, if all is due to environment, how much freedom the psychopathic individual has in choosing a behavior among others? Some answers can derive from application of epigenetics in the field, as some authors reviewed (among others, [11]). Neurobiological analysis must be completed, however, by social and developmental analysis, since it is soundly demonstrated that social and familial influences play a major role in the clinical manifestations of the disorder [12]. A new interesting and promising field of research is the opioid brain system dysfunction hypothesis; if it is confirmed, it will open new treatment models for behavioral disturbances in these patients [13].

The issue of treatment and of efficacy of treatment choices is also of extreme actuality (especially in Italy, where we are experiencing the closure of forensic asylums and the opening of forensic units governed not by justice system but by the mental health system). The first interventions focused on harm reduction (reduction of disruptive behavior to protect individuals and society), but they showed limited efficacy. Old research data suggest that treatment had low or no influence in improving the behavior of psychopaths; the same data, disappointingly, also suggest that in some cases, treatment "as usual" could worsen antisocial behavior. Persons with psychopathic structure are therefore usually considered untreatable, and an involuntary admission to a hospital (general or psychiatric) is generally not suitable. Yet psychopathy is the disorder that is most predictive of a person's future aggression and foreseeable harm to others, behaviors that are actually hardly manageable in a classical clinical context [14]. In the MacArthur study of posthospital discharge patients, a high score on psychopathy index was one of the strongest predictors of postdischarge violence (35.7% risk prevalence). Even so, the predictivity of the model was limited, as more than half of the patients with elevated psychopathy index did not express violent behavior within 6 months following discharge [15]. There is a need for efficacious treatments in order to prevent recidivism, family and social health problems, and, lastly, individual health. The issue is of particular actuality in Italy, where we have improved a massive reform closing the old asylums also in the forensic field, creating however heavy problems in terms of organization of resources, efficacy of rehabilitation programs in this specific population, influence of substance abuse on antisocial behaviors, and custodial responsibility of the criminally insane (cfr. the application of the Italian Law no. 81/2014).

Some recent reviews showed that some psychotherapeutic interventions (specifically those in cognitive-behavioral area: behavioral therapy, emotion recognition training, and multimodal interventions) early in adolescence had some chance to meliorate emotional aspects of psychopathy; on the contrary, on behavior, the usual interventions did not show a significant efficacy [16]. A recent review showed also that efficacy of interventions can modify neurobiological asset of affected individuals [17], specifically reducing activity in ventral PFC ("relaxing" effect); other effects are on hormonal axis and on heart frequency variability, with a "normalizing" effect on these parameters.

Other promising studies provide strong evidence of a strong association between CU traits and risk for poor treatment outcomes, at the same time underlining that social learning-based parent training could produce lasting improvement in CU traits, particularly when delivered early in childhood [18]. The majority of studies underline the importance of early treatment for successful outcomes [19].

Here are some final words about involuntary hospital commitment. This intervention (differently ruled across the countries but with the general structure to ensure treatments to unwilling patients) is easily justified when the unwilling patient has a mental disorder that (a) deprives him or her of the capacity to consent, (b) is amenable to psychiatric treatment, and (c) creates a serious risk of harm to himself or others. Psychopathy has undoubtedly an intrinsic high risk of harm to others (to self too, in some circumstances) but does not result in incapacity to consent, and actual psychiatric treatments, as now, have not shown adequate efficacy. Therefore, debate is still open about the efficacy and usefulness of compulsory admission in psychiatric wards of psychopaths. This debate will last for the future, unless an efficacious treatment program is developed and validated.

We should not forget also that antisocial personality disorder and psychopathy in the "real world" often does not occur in the pure state but are associated with a broad spectrum of psychiatric disorders [20]. Some of them are apparently independent (e.g., schizophrenia and mood disorders), but some of them have a dual relationship with psychopathy: in fact, substance abuse and impulsive aggression may be conceptualized as either dimensions of the basic psychopathic disturbance or considered as distinct conditions frequently cooccurring with psychopathic area disorders. In these cases, where organized, premeditated antisocial aggression predominates, pharmacotherapy alone will not modify clinical presentation of patients. According to the severity of the patient's core psychopathy, continuous postdischarge psychosocial rehabilitation and cognitive or behavioral therapy may be helpful. But even in the absence of specific and validated treatment plans, we nevertheless have to try different therapeutic approaches because a favorable response to therapeutic interventions can improve the patient's overall social functioning and decrease the risk of recidivism, even while other psychopathic traits persist.

After these short, although not exhaustive, introductive notes on psychopathy and its critical issues (not commented here are the structural dimensions of the psychopathic traits [21, 22], the neurobiology of successful vs unsuccessful psychopaths [23], or the legal, ethical, and social consequences of biological research [24]), let me introduce the present book.

The book covers some of the critical issues depicted in the preceding introductive notes, trying to give some answers according to the most updated available data.

In the first contribution, "From Moral Insanity to Psychopathy," the authors debate about the history of the nosography of psychopathy, giving some critical observations on diagnostic criteria and diagnostic tools; they also debate about some sociobiological data regarding pathogenesis of psychopathy.

In the following chapter, "Development of Psychopathy from Childhood," the author makes a broad evaluation of epidemiological, developmental, clinical, and diagnostic issues of psychopathy specifically in the early age of life.

According to the importance of early diagnosis (but also a good diagnosis) and early interventions for a good outcome of treatment, in the third chapter, "The Problem of Adolescent Psychopathy: The Downward Extension of Adult Psychopathy," the author examines some important aspects in the development of personality across different ages, differentiating personality traits (functional or dysfunctional) from personality disorders.

In the chapter "The Problem of Adolescent Psychopathy," the authors discuss the role of developmental factors from adolescence to adulthood in the stabilization process of the core features of psychopathy.

In the chapter "Cognitive Behavioral Theory and Therapy of Antisocial Personality Disorder," the author examines some new cognitive behavioral theories on the development and manifestations of antisocial personality disorder. The author, according to these new theorizations, suggests therapeutic interventions, supported by some outcome data.

The chapter "A Behavioral System Approach to Psychopathy" describes, using a strict ethological behavioral approach to the evaluation of psychopathy, the motivational dynamics underlying antisocial behavior, suggesting some specific targets of intervention.

In the seventh chapter, "The Impact of Psychopathy on the Family," to complete the picture, the author analyzes the effects of psychopathy on family members. The interesting starting point is that psychopaths are actually able to have tight bonds and are able to have a stable family (and friendship relations): their difference from "normal" is on the utilitarian scope of the bond in psychopaths. Beginning from this point of view, ethologically based, the author analyzes some relationships of psychopaths (siblings, parents, and friends) and suggests the incremental efficacy of interventions on the caregivers and not only on individuals.

In "Psychopathy: The Reflection of Severe Psychosocial Dysfunction," the author explores the different relationships of antisocial behavior, social cues and social responses to antisocial behavior, and the communicative problems of psychopaths, in order to suggest how some treatment approaches need to be better targeted in this specific population.

The last chapter covers a very intriguing issue in psychopathic functioning, the one related to "Successful Psychopaths: A Contemporary Phenomenon." The open debate, in fact, is on how psychopathic traits are widespread among successful leaders (in politics, economics, and governance in general) and how leaders' psychopathic traits affect subordinate functioning and social equilibrium as well.

Hoping in future books on the same topics, have a good reading.

Dr. Federico Durbano, MD
Director of Psychiatric Unit 34 "Martesana"
Vice Director of Mental Health and Dependences Department
ASST Melegnano e della Martesana, Italy
Contract Professor of Psychiatry at University of Milan Nursing School
Invited Professor to Criminology Master at "Il Sole 24 Ore" School of Economics

References

[1] Thompson DF, Ramos CL, Willett JK. Psychopathy: clinical features, developmental basis and therapeutic challenges. Journal of Clinical Pharmacy and Therapeutics, 2014, 39, 485–495

[2] Seara-Cardoso A, Viding E. Functional Neuroscience of Psychopathic Personality in Adults. Journal of Personality, 2015, 83:723-737

[3] Blair RJ. Psychopathy: cognitive and neural dysfunction. Dialogues in clinical neuroscience, 2013, 15:181-90

[4] Casey H, Rogers RD, Burns T, Yiend J. Emotion regulation in psychopathy. Biological Psychology, 2013, 92:541– 548

[5] Hare RD. The Revised Psychopathy Checklist. Toronto, Ontario, Canada: Multi-Health Systems, 1991.

[6] Cleckley H. The mask of sanity (5th ed.). St. Louis, MO: Mosby, 1976.

[7] Hare RD, Harpur RJ, Hakstian AR, Forth AE, Hart SD, Newman JP. The revised Psychopathology Checklist: Reliability and factor structure. Psychological Assessment, 1990, 2:338-341

[8] Harpur TJ, Hakstian AR, Hare RD. Factor structure of the Psychopathy Checklist. Journal of Consulting and Clinical Psychology, 1988, 56:741-747.

[9] Templeman R, Wong S. Determining the factor structure of the Psychopathy Checklist: A converging approach. Multivariate Experimental Clinical Research, 1994, 10:157-166.

[10] Marsh AA. Understanding amygdala responsiveness to fearful expressions through the lens of psychopathy and altruism. Journal of neuroscience research, 2016, 94:513-25

[11] Tamatea AJ. 'Biologizing' Psychopathy: Ethical, Legal, and Research Implications at the Interface of Epigenetics and Chronic Antisocial Conduct. Behav. Sci. Law, 2015, 33:629–643

[12] Piotrowska PJ, Stride CB, Croft SE, Rowe R. Socioeconomic status and antisocial behaviour among children and adolescents: A systematic review and meta-analysis. Clinical Psychology Review, 2015, 35:47-55

[13] Bandelow B, Wedekind D. Possible role of a dysregulation of the endogenous opioid system in antisocial personality disorder. Hum. Psychopharmacol Clin Exp, 2015, 30: 393–415

[14] Reidy DE, Kearns MC, DeGue S. Reducing psychopathic violence: A review of the treatment literature. Aggression and Violent Behavior, 2013, 18:527–538

[15] Monahan J, Steadman HJ, Silver E, et al. Rethinking Risk Assessment: The MacArthur Study of Mental Disorder and Violence. New York: Oxford University Press; 2001

[16] Wilkinson S, Waller R, Viding E. Practitioner Review: Involving young people with callous unemotional traits in treatment--does it work? A systematic review. Journal of child psychology and psychiatry, and allied disciplines , 2016, 57:552-65

[17] Cornet LJ, de Kogel CH, Nijman HL, Raine A, van der Laan PH. Neurobiological changes after intervention in individuals with anti-social behaviour: a literature review. Criminal behaviour and mental health: CBMH, 2015, 25:10-27
[18] Hawes DJ, Price MJ, Dadds MR. Callous-Unemotional Traits and the Treatment of Conduct Problems in Childhood and Adolescence: A Comprehensive Review. Clin Child Fam Psychol Rev, 2014, 17:248–267
[19] Salekin RT, Worley C, Grimes RD. Treatment of Psychopathy: A Review and Brief Introduction to the Mental Model Approach for Psychopathy. Behav. Sci. Law, 2010, 28:235–266
[20] Glenn AL, Johnson AK, Raine A. Antisocial Personality Disorder: A Current Review. Curr Psychiatry Rep, 2013, 15:427-435
[21] Marcus DK, Fulton JJ, Edens JF. The Two-Factor Model of Psychopathic Personality: Evidence from the Psychopathic Personality Inventory. Personality Disorders, 2013, 4:67-76
[22] Lilienfeld SO, Watts AL, Smith SF, Berg JM, Latzman RD. Psychopathy Deconstructed and Reconstructed: Identifying and Assembling the Personality Building Blocks of Cleckley's Chimera. Journal of Personality, 2015, 83:593-610
[23] Gao Y, Raine A. Successful and Unsuccessful Psychopaths: A Neurobiological Model. Behav. Sci. Law, 2010, 28: 194–210
[24] Tamatea AJ. 'Biologizing' Psychopathy: Ethical, Legal, and Research Implications at the Interface of Epigenetics and Chronic Antisocial Conduct. Behav. Sci. Law, 2015, 33: 629–643

Chapter 1

From Moral Insanity to Psychopathy

Liliana Lorettu, Alessandra M. Nivoli and
Giancarlo Nivoli

Additional information is available at the end of the chapter

http://dx.doi.org/10.5772/intechopen.69013

Abstract

Psychopathy is currently a condition that arouses great interest among psychiatrists because of its significant involvement in the forensic field. The authors illustrate the course over time of the concept of psychopathy, starting from the definition of "moral insanity" of Prichard. The historical journey allows to illustrate the different positions that the various European schools of psychiatry have had toward psychopathy, until modern nosographic classification systems such as Diagnostic and Statistical Manual of Mental Disorders (DSM). Special attention is paid to the "core" of psychopathy: the alteration of the moral sense, and through the illustration of moral development is provided a reading of morality in the psychopath and the reasons for its impairment. A clinical and critical examination of psychopathy assessment scales is proposed, with the aim to broaden the horizons of assessment, also to individuals who do not show violent behavior, but with compromised moral sense. Lastly, authors propose an interpretation of the social aspects of psychopathy that goes beyond the assessment of the psychopath confined in jails, with several highlighted aspects of psychopathy that contribute to social success in work, relationships, and career and that can contribute to the success of the psychopath.

Keywords: psychopathy, moral insanity, psychopathology of morality, clinical features, successful of psychopathy

1. Introduction

The psychopathic syndrome is arguably one of the most dangerous and controversial constellations of personality traits, and has significant clinical and social importance. The syndrome of psychopathy has been described differently over time by a number of authors and scientific societies; despite these differences, all definitions of psychopathy highlight the impairment of the psychopath's moral capacity. This chapter addresses the following key themes: psychopathology of morality, clinical features of psychopathy, psychopathy as a diagnostic entity, and social aspects of psychopathy.

2. Background

In the early 1800s, psychiatrists began to focus their attention on individuals who displayed particularly cruel and violent forms of behavior without suffering from any clear mental pathology.

In 1809, Pinel [1] introduced the term "partial insanity" or "mania without delusion" (*manie sans délire*) to denote a condition in which "no sensible alteration of the intellect, perception, judgment, imagination, or memory is observed, but there is a perversion of the affective functions, a blind impulse to violent acts…where it is not possible to identify any dominant idea or illusion of the imagination as a determining cause of this baleful trend."

Esquirol [2] later labeled as "affective and impulsive monomania" alterations of the will that exist independently of any alteration of ideas, affecting individuals who "do not rave and ramble, whose ideas maintain their natural links, whose reasoning is logical, whose speech is not only coherent but often lively and witty, but whose actions are opposed to their affects, their interests and social custom. Their actions are irrational in the sense that they oppose their own habits and those of the people with whom they live. However disordered their actions, these monomaniacs always have more or less plausible reasons to justify themselves, so that one can say they are reasoning madmen."

The term "moral insanity" was introduced by Prichard [3] to describe a "madness consisting in a morbid perversion of the natural feelings, affections, inclinations, temper, habits, moral dispositions, and natural impulses, without any remarkable disorder or defect of the interest or knowing and reasoning faculties, and particularly without any insane illusion or hallucinations." "In cases of this description the moral and active principles of the mind are strangely perverted and depraved; the power of self-government is lost or greatly impaired; and the individual is found to be incapable, not of talking or reasoning upon any subject proposed to him, for this he will often do with great shrewdness and volubility, but of conducting himself with decency and propriety in the business of life."

Morel [4] defined "moral insanity" as "a delirium of feelings and actions with preservation of the intellectual faculties," and he asserted the hereditary basis and degenerative nature of the affliction.

The psychiatrists of the time were not unanimous in the definition and description of the clinical picture, and a debate colored by the orientations of different schools of thought soon ensued and dragged on over time.

While there was a general consensus on the description of the clinical picture, two questions became the focus of attention and the site for clashes among different schools of thought.

1. Whether the clinical manifestation was acquired or congenital.
2. Whether it was an autonomous "psychopathological syndrome" or a manifestation/symptom of more complex psychopathological syndromes.

In Italy, there were diverse interpretive frameworks: some viewed moral insanity as "a form of madness distinct and independent from other forms" and others as "a simple variety or degree of common forms of madness." Verga [5] distinguished moral insanity from monomania and defined both as "acquired frenzies."

Levi [6] attributed a congenital character to moral insanity and argued for a differential diagnosis between monomania and moral insanity. He affirmed that monomania "compels the sufferer with a blind, automatic, and irresistible impulse—sometimes against the person's conscience and will—to commit a given action, often a crime." In moral insanity, on the other hand, "the person is led to commit immoral, wicked and cruel acts of all kinds, not as a result of a special instinctive impetus … but as a result of an actual paralysis of the moral sense, which renders the intellect blind to the ideas of good and evil and dull to the feelings of shame and remorse." By contrast, Bini [7] maintained that moral insanity was not an autonomous pathological entity but a "variety" of other pathologies.

With regard to the congenital or acquired nature of moral insanity, the Italian school, in particular Tanzi [8] and Lombroso [9], tended to maintain that the clinical picture arose congenitally, and moral insanity came to be defined as a "constitutional anomaly."

However, in the early twentieth century, moral insanity and monomania lost their status as diagnosable disorders and were merged into the psychopathological descriptions of other mental conditions.

Kraepelin's contributions to psychiatry [10] constituted a milestone in the field: He moved away from the concept of *single psychosis* and instead identified two broad groups of mental pathology: *dementia praecox* and *manic depressive psychosis.*

He also linked the concept of mental illness to an organic basis: an underlying brain injury was the cause of the mental disorder.

Kraepelin moreover replaced Koch's concept of "psychopathic inferiority" with the definition of "psychopathic states," that is, conditions that affect individuals with certain distinctive personality traits. From that moment onward, the adjective "psychopathic" became associated with the noun "personality," and the concept of psychopathic personalities started to gain ground.

Thus from the early 1900s, German psychiatry brought together under the heading of psychopathy the old French diagnosis of "moral insanity" and current personality disorders.

Arieti [11] described two distinct types of psychopaths:

- The simple psychopath, characterized by an epicurean lifestyle, poor introspective skills, aggressive behavior, the pursuit of privileges, and pursuit of the pleasure principle at the expense of the reality principle;

- The complex psychopath, distinguished by lack of impulsiveness, coldness of feeling, and the ability to manipulate and exploit others.

Later, the DSM would describe personality disorders, and in its different editions, it would adopt a variety of positions toward psychopathy.

However, the debate about whether psychopathy can constitute a diagnosis remains open to this day.

3. Psychopathology of morality

All definitions of psychopathy highlight the impairment of the psychopath's moral capacity, and indeed the definition that preceded the concept of psychopathy was, for a long time, that of "moral insanity." Thus, in order to understand psychopathy better, it is useful to delve more deeply into the development of the moral sense in individuals from childhood to adulthood.

Despite their diversity of opinions, researchers agree on two things: the first is that the development of morality takes place in successive stages, and the second is that the earliest years of life play a crucial role not only in personality formation, but also in social behavior. It follows that adult personality is an expression of characteristics developed during childhood also with regard to morality.

Piaget [12] was one of the first psychologists to focus on children's morality. He tried to understand their concept of good and evil by analyzing children's play. Observing the rules of children's games and using interviews about such behaviors as stealing and lying, Piaget found that morality can be understood as a developmental process. Children's earliest sense of morality is based on strict adherence to rules, duties, and obedience to authority: it is firmly linked to the conviction that a wrong action is automatically followed by punishment.

Subsequently, moral development is based on interaction with other children, and the discovery that strict adherence to rules can itself be problematic. Thus, a transition to a new stage becomes necessary. At this point, children develop a stage of autonomous moral thinking characterized by two elements: a critical and selective capacity to interpret rules, and an appreciation of mutual respect and cooperation. Piaget concluded that this autonomous morality, which takes into account the respect of others, is more solid and leads to more coherent behaviors than the moral sense of younger children.

Kohlberg [13, 14] later developed a theory of moral development that comprises six stages (**Table 1**).

Kohlberg's theory maintains that during childhood, conduct is governed by the first two developmental stages, in which morality is conditioned by punishment and obedience, as well as individualism and exchange.

Later moral stages are reached through a process of social learning that is conditioned, among other things, by the environment surrounding the individual's everyday life. The moral criteria that are thus acquired from the familial and social context will continue into adulthood.

Stage	Behavior
Premorality	
Stage 1—Punishment and obedience orientation	Obedience to rules with the aim of avoiding punishment (similar to Piaget's first stage)
Stage 2—Individualism and exchange	Adjustment to rules in order to gain rewards or benefits
Conventional morality	
Stage 3—Morality as a means to maintain good relations with others and win their approval	Compliance with rules in order to maintain good relations with others and avoid their disapproval
Stage 4—Maintenance of the social order	Compliance with rules in order to avoid censure from the authorities
Morality as acceptance of moral principles	
Stage 5—Morality of the social contract, individual rights, and widely accepted and shared laws	Desire to maintain a properly functioning society (although the question of what constitutes a "good" society is first raised at this point)
Stage 6—Universal principles	Morality based on individual principles of conscience
	Individual's compliance with his or her own principles in order to avoid contrition

Table 1. Kohlberg's theory of moral development.

The highest level of moral reasoning, defined as post-conventional, is the level at which the individual follows universal ethical principles that may not necessarily be in accord with the law, but which answer to the individual's own conscience.

Further studies carried out in the 1970s brought a critical contribution to Kohlberg's theory of moral development. In particular, it is fruitful to recall the contributions of Turiel [15] and Gilligan [16].

Turiel's studies led to the formulation of domain theory.

This theory holds that children as young as 39 months of age already have two different conceptual domains that regulate morality: one domain is of external origin, namely social conventions, while the other has an intrinsic origin and corresponds to moral imperatives. The two domains have different effects, so that transgressing conventions is considered less serious than disobeying universally recognized moral norms.

On the other hand, Gilligan has developed a concept of great contemporary relevance, namely the idea that morality consists in care rather than justice or rights. There is thus a sort of moral obligation to solidarity rather than an obligation not to wrong others.

With regard to psychopaths, Kohlberg [13] was the first to find that young people with antisocial behavior displayed pre-conventional moral reasoning, which suggests that there has been an arrest in moral development, influenced in part by negative life experiences.

Later, Campagna and Harter [17] used interviews based on Kohlberg's method to examine the differences in moral reasoning that distinguished a group of **young psychopaths** from a control group.

The study revealed that psychopaths exhibited a lower level of moral reasoning than the control group of the same mental age. Among psychopaths, moral reasoning was predominantly at the pre-conventional stage, whereas the control group followed conventional modes of moral reasoning appropriate to their age. The members of the control group displayed types of moral reasoning that went beyond individual needs to take into account the social context and shared norms. The moral reasoning of psychopaths was instead rooted in an egocentric position focused on the individual's own needs and the balance between anticipated gain and risks incurred by their actions.

Other studies have confirmed that psychopaths exhibit a level of moral reasoning similar to that of children under the age of 10, falling under the pre-conventional stage in Kohlberg's scale [17–23].

At this point, the question that arises is: why do psychopaths display levels of moral reasoning lower than those of normal subjects? Are environmental influences and negative life experiences sufficient to account for this arrest in moral development?

Kohlberg's hypothesis on the development of moral reasoning also takes into consideration the processes of cognitive development, postulating a parallelism between cognitive development and the development of moral reasoning. From this perspective, the maturation of complex cognitive structures is considered a necessary condition and a prerequisite for progressing through the various developmental stages of moral reasoning.

This hypothesis is buttressed by a study performed by Campagna and Harter [17], in which a group of psychopathic subjects and a control group were tested using the Wechsler Intelligence Scale for Children. The study showed that children who attained higher scores in cognitive intelligence also exhibited higher levels of moral reasoning.

This result lends credence to the hypothesis of a link between the cognitive system and its development, on the one hand, and the development of moral reasoning, on the other, such that impairment in the latter would be correlated with a deficient cognitive system.

According to the hypothesis, both systems would be impaired in psychopaths.

This hypothesis could constitute the key to interpret a number of cases of psychopathy that display both impairment of moral reasoning and cognitive deficits. However, actual clinical cases are more complex and nuanced: it is often possible to encounter psychopaths who display a good intellectual level of development, sometimes even higher than average, who employ their intelligence to achieve their personal goals through the manipulation of others.

Other authors have reported, through brain-imaging studies, that the brains of psychopaths exhibit differences from those of normal subjects in the orbital cortex, which deals with ethical thought, moral choices, and impulse control [24]. Other researchers have found that the experience of violence as a source of pleasure or displeasure is associated with the functioning of the nucleus accumbens [25].

On the other hand, psychological theories have long emphasized that insecure attachment and trauma are closely linked with antisocial and violent behavior [26–28].

Meloy's position [29] synthesizes the complexity of these arguments. He asserts: "My theoretical and clinical hypothesis is that psychopathy is psychobiologically predisposed, but there are necessarily deficient and conflictual primary object experiences that determine its phenotypic expression."

Despite its theoretical appeal as well as its partial truth and clinical applicability, this position leaves unanswered the question that was initially posed back in the nineteenth century by the first scholars who described moral insanity and later psychopathy. Even after so much time has elapsed, it is still not easy to provide an exhaustive answer today, although there is a general consensus that psychopathy is an early onset pervasive personality disorder. Yet the question of how the various biological, psychological, and relational "etiologies" affect the "moral core" remains a mystery to be unraveled.

4. Clinical features of psychopathy

Many authors have described the clinical features of psychopathy, but Cleckley's [30, 31] clinical description stands out among others and constitutes a milestone. In his book "The Mask of Sanity," Cleckley sorts through observations from a wide range of cases in order to identify 16 specific traits that characterize psychopaths (**Table 2**).

1. Considerable superficial charm and average or above average intelligence
2. Absence of delusions and other signs of irrational thinking
3. Absence of anxiety or other "neurotic" symptoms. Considerable poise, calmness, and verbal facility
4. Unreliability, disregard for obligations, no sense of responsibility, in matters of little and great import
5. Untruthfulness and insincerity
6. Antisocial behavior which is inadequately motivated and poorly planned, seeming to stem from an inexplicable impulsiveness
7. Inadequately motivated antisocial behavior
8. Poor judgment and failure to learn from experience
9. Pathological egocentricity. Total self-centeredness and an incapacity for real love and attachment
10. General poverty of deep and lasting emotions
11. Lack of any true insight; inability to see oneself as others do
12. Ingratitude for any special considerations, kindness, and trust
13. Fantastic and objectionable behavior, after drinking and sometimes even when not drinking. Vulgarity, rudeness, quick mood shifts, pranks for facile entertainment
14. No history of genuine suicide attempts
15. An impersonal, trivial, and poorly integrated sex life
16. Failure to have a life plan and to live in an ordered way (unless it is for destructive purposes or a sham)

Table 2. Hervey Cleckley's list of psychopathy symptoms.

The clinical features of these patients can be traced back not only to their behavior, but also to the style of their interpersonal relationships and their affective lives. These 16 traits highlight the absence of any psychopathological alterations; indeed, Cleckley describes psychopaths as endowed with charm and intelligence, not suffering from delusions or irrational thinking, without "nervousness" or psychoneurotic symptoms (traits 1–3). Instead, the list underlines aspects, such as the subjects' ability to present a false representation of reality (traits 4 and 5), and peculiarities of their affective life, such as lack of remorse or shame, the inability to learn from experience, egocentricity and the inability to love, a significant poverty in major emotional reactions, and callousness in interpersonal relationships (traits 6, 8, 9, 10, and 12). There are also purely behavioral aspects such as the lack of adequate motivation for antisocial behavior, the display of bizarre behaviors, promiscuous and impersonal sexual behavior, and the inability to take up a life project (traits 7, 12, 13, and 16). The whole is accompanied by a distinctive lack of insight (trait 11).

Hare [32, 33] later developed the Psychopathy Checklist (PCL) (**Table 3**) as a tool for clinical evaluation of an individual's degree of psychopathy through the use of a semi-structured

1. Glibness/superficial charm
2. Grandiose sense of self-worth
3. Need for stimulation/proneness to boredom
4. Pathological lying
5. Cunning/manipulative
6. Lack of remorse or guilt
7. Shallow affect
8. Callousness/lack of empathy
9. Parasitic lifestyle
10. Poor behavioral controls
11. Promiscuous sexual behavior
12. Early behavior problems
13. Lack of realistic long-term goals
14. Impulsivity
15. Irresponsibility
16. Failure to accept responsibility for own actions
17. Many short-term marital relationships
18. Juvenile delinquency
19. Revocation of conditional release
20. Criminal versatility

Table 3. Hare's psychopathy checklist.

interview along with information obtained from the individual, his or her family members, and police reports.

The PCL-R consists of 20 items that fall into two main groups:

- The first, referred to as factor 1 and labeled as affective/interpersonal deficit, describes a subject with inflated self-esteem, selfish, without remorse, and exploitative of others;
- The second, known as factor 2, identifies an antisocial lifestyle characterized by impulsivity and irresponsibility.

In subsequent studies, based on the analysis of latent variables [34], Hare supported the four-factor PCL-R model. This model measures four dimensions of psychopathy that are strongly interrelated: interpersonal, affective, lifestyle, and antisocial. Factor 1 scores the individual's interpersonal dimension and comprises four items (glibness, grandiose sense of self-worth, pathological lying, and manipulation). Factor 2 scores emotional responses and quality of relations with others and comprises four items (lack of remorse or guilt, shallow affect, lack of empathy, and failure to accept responsibility). Factor 3 refers to the individual's lifestyle and comprises five items (need for constant stimulation/proneness to boredom, parasitic lifestyle, lack of realistic goals, impulsivity, and irresponsibility). Factor 4 measures antisocial behaviors and has five items (poor behavior controls, early behavior problems, juvenile delinquency, revocation of conditional release, and criminal versatility).

Meloy [29] stresses that the main characteristics of psychopaths relate to their affective lives, which lack emotional ties, key reference figures, and emotional involvement in actions. Thus, psychopaths are able to commit the most cruel and brutal acts without hesitation, with emotional coldness, and without concern for the consequences that might befall them or their victims. The psychopath is a "lone wolf" who, unlike the antisocial individual, does not adhere to criminal subcultures, since the psychopath is unable to establish personal ties or follow rules, be they the rules of society or of a criminal underworld.

Another distinctive aspect of psychopaths is their capacity for seduction. Hare has drawn attention to this aspect in his description of the typical conversation with a psychopath, which is often rich in details, half-truths, fragments of speech, and internal contradictions. It is not a type of conversation from which useful information can be gained, but it is rather marked by the psychopath's deployment of charm, seduction, and manipulation.

Through their allure, seductiveness, and clever use of lying, psychopaths are expert manipulators of those around them.

Psychopaths may in fact be defined as "intra-species predators who use charm, manipulation, violence, intimidation, and a constant violation of other's rights in order to control them and satisfy their own egoistical needs" [35, 36].

Hare divided psychopathy into three different categories:

1. "Primary" or "true" psychopaths. These individuals are not characterized by violence and/or destructiveness. Rather, they are characterized by sociality, glibness, and charm. They are apparently normal, calm, and collected. The crux of psychopathy in their case

consists in their being unable to feel any emotion, and in their extraordinary ability to manipulate and seduce. They are extremely skilled individuals, so much so that they rarely get caught by the criminal justice system and, when they do, they often fare well thanks to their manipulation skills.

2. The second category is that of "secondary" or "neurotic" psychopaths. These individuals display particularly cruel and heinous violent behavior without feelings of guilt or remorse. They have difficulty managing their emotions and are often impulsive. They often commit crimes, and often get arrested.

3. Hare's third category is that of "dyssocial" psychopaths. These individuals are driven to acts that deviate from the social environment to which they belong, following dysfunctional models learned from significant figures in their lives. They differ from other psychopaths in that they have the capacity to experience guilt and to establish affective relationships. Hare claims that Bandura's social learning theory could provide a key to understanding the behavior of dissocial psychopaths, explaining how their behavior stems from their culture and the society that surrounds them [37].

On the other hand, Millon and Davis [38] propose a classification of ten types of psychopathy based on character traits, behavioral aspects, and defence mechanisms. Their classification was partly taken up in the Psychodynamic Diagnostic Manual (PDM, 2006), which distinguishes between two subgroups of psychopaths: the first includes aggressive, explosive, predatory, and violent psychopaths, while the second comprises less aggressive individuals devoted to a parasitic and dependent lifestyle based on fraud.

From Cleckley onward, and subsequently with Hare, clinical descriptions of psychopathy have tended to approach it as a dimension involving a great variety of clinical manifestations.

However, certain limitations are worth noting.

PCL-R has proved to be a useful tool for diagnosing psychopathy and for differentiating it from Antisocial Personality Disorder (ASPD).

The first limitation is inherent in this clinical scale and stems from its origin: PCL-R, like Cleckley's checklist before it, was developed from the observation of violent offenders; consequently, this scale reflects specifically those individuals but risks leaving out many false negatives: people who have not committed violent offences, yet are psychopaths insofar as their moral sense is deeply impaired and this affects their behavior and relationships. PCL-R measures the maladaptive characteristics of psychopathy and would seem to be biased toward a specific subgroup of psychopaths, that is, violent ones. Consequently, a large number of psychopaths risk remaining unrecognized.

Moreover, although studies have shown a high level of interrater reliability, rater training may differ, leading to contradictory assessments [39].

The second limitation concerns another use of PCL-R, which is to assess the risk of violence. PCL-R is considered an important tool in violence risk assessment; specifically, it belongs to several actuarial tools for measuring the risk of violence, such as HCR-20 (Historical Clinical and Risk Management) and VRAG (Violence Risk Appraisal Guide). However, a recent article has highlighted the limitations of violence risk assessment tools on account of the many false positives and false negatives which risk "distorting" treatment and social policy interventions, but especially because they are weak outcome indicators in terms of actual reduction in violence [40].

5. Psychopathy as a diagnostic entity

5.1. Psychopathy and the DSM

The construct of psychopathy has had a troubled, and at times controversial, relationship with the American Psychiatric Association's (APA) Diagnostic and Statistical Manual of Mental Disorders (DSM).

The ***DSM-I*** [41] included a category termed "sociopathic personality disturbance," one subcategory of which was "antisocial reaction." These individuals were defined as "chronically antisocial," and as profiting from neither experience nor punishment; they maintained no real loyalties to any person and were "frequently callous and hedonistic," with a lack of any sense of responsibility. The definition included all cases previously classified as "constitutional psychopathic state" and "psychopathic personality."

The ***DSM-II*** [42] defined the "antisocial personality" using clinical criteria closer to Cleckley's definition of psychopathy (**Table 2**), indicating that these persons were "grossly selfish, callous, irresponsible, impulsive, and unable to feel guilt or to learn from experience and punishment," in addition to being drawn "repeatedly into conflict with society," having low frustration tolerance and having a tendency to blame others for their problems. Based on this definition, a mere history of repeated legal or social offences was not sufficient to justify diagnosis. Despite its importance, Cleckley's work did not propose a standardized method to evaluate or measure the clinical features identified, and thus remained confined to the field of pure theory.

A significant shift came about with the ***DSM-III*** [43], whose major innovation consisted in the inclusion of specific and explicit criterion sets [44]. Feighner et al. [45] developed specific and explicit criterion sets for 14 mental disorders, and Antisocial Personality Disorder (ASPD) was the only personality disorder included. The inclusion of ASPD in Feighner et al. [45] was due largely to Robins' [46] systematic study of "sociopathic" personality disorder, closely linked to Cleckley's concept of psychopathy. Robins included a number of key Cleckley traits, such as lack of guilt, pathological lying, and the use of aliases (without including other items such as the lack of a sense of shame, the inability to accept blame, and to learn from experience, egocentricity, inadequate depth of feeling, and lack of insight). In addition, Robins' list contained other nonspecific dysfunctions such as somatic complaints, suicide attempts or risk, drug use, and problems with alcohol consumption. Most of Robins' items were accompanied by quite specific requirements for their assessment. For example, the determination of a poor marital history required "two or more divorces, marriage to wives with severe behaviour problems, repeated separations"; the category of repeated arrests was described as "three or more non-traffic arrests"; and an assessment of impulsive behavior required "frequent moving from one city to another, more than one elopement, sudden army enlistments or unprovoked desertion of home" [46]. Robins' 19-item list [46] was reduced by Feighner et al. [45] to 9 items, including conduct disorder (required), along with poor work history, irresponsible parenting, unlawful behavior, relationship infidelity or instability, aggressiveness, financial irresponsibility, lack of regard for the truth, and recklessness [43].

New to the ***DSM-III-R*** criterion set was the item "lacks remorse," obtained from the PCL and Cleckley, along with impulsivity or failure to plan ahead [47]. A related criticism of the DSM-III criterion set was that it placed too much emphasis on a particular type of behavior, namely criminality [48]. "The DSM-III criteria set may have selected too many criminals and excluded persons who were not criminal but who demonstrated the social irresponsibility, lack of guilt, disloyalty, lack of empathy, and exploitation central to most theories of psychopathy" [49]. However, the development of the DSM-III coincided with the development of the Psychopathy Checklist (PCL) by Hare [32]. The PCL included Cleckley's traits of superficial charm, lack of remorse, egocentricity, and lack of emotional depth, none of which were included in DSM-III. On the other hand, the PCL did not include a number of the traits identified by Cleckley, for example, absence of delusions, good intelligence, fantastic behavior with drink, and suicide.

The ***DSM-IV*** [50] took into consideration a revised version of the PCL, the PCL-R, which included the deletion of two items (drug and alcohol abuse, and a prior diagnosis of psychopathy) and the broadening of the irresponsibility item to involve domains beyond simply parenting. The diagnostic criteria associated with ASPD in the DSM-IV were related to the failure to conform to social norms, deceitfulness, impulsivity, irritability and aggressiveness, reckless disregard for safety of self or others, and consistent irresponsibility.

By the time of the ***DSM-5*** [51], there was considerably more research concerning psychopathy than ASPD [52]. The authors of the DSM-5 referred to a new hybrid model of psychopathy developed concurrently with the DSM-5: the triarchic model of psychopathy, assessed with the Triarchic Psychopathy Measure (TriPM), by Patrick et al. [53]. These authors identified three elements they considered essential to the understanding of psychopathy: boldness, meanness, and disinhibition. Further revisions made to the proposed criterion set for ASPD included three additional traits as potential specifiers for psychopathy: low anxiousness, low social withdrawal, and high attention-seeking [51]. In any case, the proposed diagnostic criteria are not different from those of the DSM-IV-tr (**Table 4**).

The psychopathic syndrome is probably one of the most dangerous and virulent constellations of personality traits, and it has significant clinical and social importance. The syndrome of psychopathy has been described differently by a number of authors and scientific societies [30–33, 41–43, 46, 47, 50–56]. There is "a lack of consensus regarding its conceptualization," and it has been suggested that existing descriptions may be alternative constructions of the same hypothetical entity [48, 57]. The choice of which particular constellation to use in research or clinical practice is perhaps best made on the basis of which proves to be most useful for social or clinical purposes or, at best, which represents the consensus view within the field.

http://dx.doi.org/10.5772/intechopen.69013

A. There is a pervasive pattern of disregard for, and violation of, the rights of others, occurring since age 15, as indicated by three (or more) of the following:

1. Failure to conform to social norms with respect to lawful behaviors, as indicated by repeatedly performing acts that are grounds for arrest
2. eceitfulness, as indicated by repeated lying, use of aliases, or conning others for personal profit or pleasure
3. Impulsivity or failure to plan ahead
4. Irritability and aggressiveness, as indicated by repeated physical fights or assaults
5. Reckless disregard for the safety of self or others
6. Consistent irresponsibility, as indicated by being indifferent to or rationalizing having hurt, mistreated, or stolen from others

B. The individual is at least 18 years of age

C. There is evidence of conduct disorder with onset before age 15

D. Antisocial behavior does not occur exclusively during a schizophrenic or manic episode

Table 4. DSM-5 criteria for antisocial personality disorder.

6. Social aspects of psychopathy

It is common to find dysfunctional psychopaths in prison, involved in more or less complex legal proceedings and caught up in scarcely enviable criminal careers. Indeed, many studies of psychopathy are born from the observation of incarcerated individuals. Cleckley studied a significant number of such individuals and made an important contribution to the clinical description of psychopathy. Nevertheless, the title that he gave to his work, "The Mask of Sanity," suggests that we should observe psychopathy in a more articulated way.

It is likely that the social aspects of psychopathy, that is, the imprint that the condition leaves on an individual's lifestyle and quality of life, are more complex and multifaceted than those we typically tend to observe.

Evaluation of the social aspects of psychopathy has long been affected by two gross biases: a limited observational perspective and the observer's "countertransference" (understood in the broadest sense as the evaluator's total set of emotional reactions).

With regard to the first bias, the observational perspective has often relied on incarcerated individuals; hence, what was observed was the dysfunctional effect of psychopathy on the lives of these individuals, whose lives were spent in prison or at any rate in the grip of the judicial system.

However, close observation of the real world would find numerous psychopaths whose lives have "benefited" from certain elements of psychopathy. Many successful psychopaths occupy prestigious positions in politics, finance, and entertainment.

Keeping in mind that the lack of morality is a constant element of psychopathy, it is useful to examine critically certain other elements of this condition and evaluate their positive or negative effect in terms of positioning the psychopath among either dysfunctional or successful individuals.

Dysfunctional elements notably include impulsivity, the recourse to violence, and poor judgment.

Impulsivity is dysfunctional because it is a very primordial element that leads to action without prior evaluation of consequences or of the situation's complexity: impulsivity is no ally to developing tactics or strategies, or to social functioning.

The recourse to violence has always been associated with psychopathy. Numerous psychopaths are authors of particularly cruel and heinous violent acts. They are capable of committing such abhorrent acts because their feelings are anaesthetized, so they can act with coldness. Violent behavior is often committed as the result of impulsivity and without calculation of the consequences for the perpetrator or the victim. The use of violence is a dysfunctional element because it inevitably leads to the psychopath's confrontation with the judicial system, leading to consequences such as imprisonment and the restriction of freedom.

The poor judgment displayed by psychopaths has led to their being considered cognitively deficient. Indeed, some psychopaths exhibit forms of intellectual impairment that have played an important role in the dysfunctionality that marks their lives.

On the other hand, the elements that play a role in the social success of some psychopaths include seductiveness, coldness of feeling, the role of empathy, emotional resilience, and the ability to manipulate others.

Even dysfunctional psychopaths display some charm and seductive abilities, albeit only superficially and in a relatively more recognizable manner. By contrast, charm and seductiveness are the signature traits of the successful psychopath. These individuals' allure is complemented by a high and sometimes remarkable intelligence, which enables them to easily conquer their prey.

Indeed, these individuals' charm relies on their capacity to manipulate others. Thanks to their loquacity, psychopaths can be extremely skillful manipulators who do not hesitate to deploy lies or half-truths and present them as universal and irrefutable facts. They thus manage to make others see a partial view of reality and to persuade them in ways that ultimately lead to the psychopath's own personal gain.

For a long time, the psychopath was described as an individual incapable of feeling empathy. This is only true in respect of a limited concept of empathy as the ability to understand the feelings of another or the ability to "put oneself in the other's shoes."

It is however necessary to "broaden" the concept of empathy in order to understand the psychopath. Studies on mirror neurons show that empathy also exists in the animal world [58, 59], and it is precisely the animal world that helps us better understand the psychopath. Thanks to a complex sensory system, animals are able to grasp when certain things are about to happen; for instance, an animal can understand that a predator is approaching, even without seeing the attacker, because it feels the latter's presence through a set of "signs." Some animals are also capable of sensing disruptive weather events, for example, the arrival of a thunderstorm, even before the appearance of any clear signal heralding the event. Psychopaths operate in a way that is very similar to the evolutionary system that gives animals protection. While it is true that psychopaths do not experience empathy in the sense that they are completely indifferent to the mood and suffering of others, it would be a grave mistake to think that they do not understand the emotions of others: in fact, psychopaths have an innate and extraordinary capacity to read and understand emotions, and to exploit them to their advantage.

Moreover, the psychopath has considerable emotional resilience. Resilience is a concept derived from physics that describes a material's capacity to resist external traumatic force.

In psychology, resilience refers to the capacity to cope with traumatic events in a positive way. The psychopaths' emotional resilience corresponds to their capacity to overcome any difficulties related to, or derived from, emotions in order to focus solely on their own personal gain. Thus, psychopaths allow neither the emotions of others nor their own to obstruct their path; they are deaf and blind to feelings and pay heed only to their own pleasure.

Emotional resilience in fact accounts for the low level of anxiety that is present in the successful psychopath. Anxiety, like fear, does not belong in the psychopath's emotional makeup. Freedom from anxiety in turn facilitates the psychopath's riskiest behaviors; not suffering from anxiety or fear, the psychopath tackles risk where normal individuals would be thwarted by fear. The ability to face risk, which resolves in a form of courage, gives the psychopath access to higher chances of success than would be possible for an individual with a timid or fearful attitude.

Additionally, the psychopath's grandiose self-esteem reinforces his courage and emotional resilience.

The successful psychopath also uses violence, but it is rarely the kind of brutal and heinous physical violence that would cause the perpetrator's immediate identification, labeling, and exclusion. Instead, the successful psychopath is an extraordinary master of psychological violence, which he uses in the manipulation of others. The victim of psychological violence often does not recognize it as such because the psychopath's charm and manipulative ability render it extremely difficult to identify his/her psychological aggressions.

The foregoing considerations, which spring from empirical, clinical observations, are confirmed by recent publications that highlight the positive aspects of psychopathy and suggest the possibility that these elements at times serve as sources of success in business, at work, and in relationships [60]. These considerations also suggest that certain aspects of psychopathy are more widespread in the general population than was thought, and are not confined to the prison population [61].

The other element that can lead to errors in the evaluation of psychopaths is "countertransference," understood as a therapist's full range of emotional reactions toward a patient. The therapist may deploy defence mechanisms such as identification with the victim, identification with the aggressor, projection, projective identification, etc., which often create obstacles to a correct diagnostic evaluation [62]. When dealing with psychopaths, the therapist's perception may be further distorted by his/her moral judgment. Whether dysfunctional or successful, the psychopath exhibits moral impairment; often, in fact, the first observation that a therapist makes, even before further assessment, is that the individual appears to be amoral. This results in a counter-transferential conditioning that prevents the evaluator from seeing the psychopath's social success, and when social success is recognized, this recognition precludes detection of the individual's psychopathic traits.

In conclusion, the conceptualization of psychopathy should move away from a vision of the psychopath as a sort of Hannibal Lecter. Though in some cases true, this vision is not the only applicable model; a different model that stands worlds apart but belongs also to the psychopathic dimension is that of a respected and successful head of government.

Psychopathy is increasingly understood as a spectrum disorder, with highly differentiated qualitative and quantitative expressions. This variability holds even for single traits so that, for example, one could have impulsivity at one end and the ability to act deliberately at the other, with widely different results along the spectrum.

Hence, the great dilemma that we sometimes grapple with in the face of an individual—mad or bad?—becomes more complex in the face of the psychopath—dysfunctional or successful?

Author details

Liliana Lorettu*, Alessandra M. Nivoli and Giancarlo Nivoli

*Address all correspondence to: lloretu@uniss.it

Psychiatric Clinica, Department of Clinical and Experimental Medicine,
University of Sassari, Italy

References

[1] Pinel P. Traité médico phylosophique sur l'aliénation mentale ou la manie. Paris: Brosson; 1809

[2] Esquirol JED. Des passions considerées comme causes, symptôms et moyenes curatifs de l'aliénation mentale. Paris: Didot; 1802

[3] Prichard JC. A Treatise on Insanity and Other Disorders Affecting the Mind. London: Sherwood Gilbert, a. Piper; 1835

[4] Morel BA. Traité des maladies mentales. Paris: Masson; 1860

[5] Verga A. Monomania Istintiva. Milano: Gazzetta Medica Lombardi; 1849

[6] Levi C. Della monomania in relazione col Foro criminale. Rivista Sperimentale di Freniatria. 1876;**2**:394,639

[7] Bini F. Definizione e classificazione delle pazzie. Archivio Italiano Malattie Nervose. 1879;**16**:210

[8] Tanzi E. Pazzi morali e delinquenti nati. Rivista sperimentale di Freniatria. 1884;**10**:266

[9] Lombroso C. Identità dell'epilessia colla pazzia morale e delinquenza congenita. Achivi di Psichiatria, Scienze Penali e Antropologia Criminale. 1885;**6**:1

[10] Kraepelin E. Compendio di Psichiatria. Napoli: Vallardi; 1885

[11] Arieti S. Trattato di Psichiatria. Milano: Boringhieri; 1985

[12] Piaget J. Il giudizio morale nel fanciullo. Firenze: Giunti Barbera; 1972

[13] Kohlberg L. The development of modes of moral thinking and choice in the years ten to sixteen [Unpublished doctoral dissertation]. University of Chicago; 1958

[14] Kohlberg L. Stage and sequence: The cognitive-developmental approach to socialization. In Goslin DA, editor. Handbook of Socialization Theory and Research. Chicago, IL: Rand McNally; 1969

[15] Turiel E. The Development of Social Knowledge: Morality and Convention. Cambridge: Cambridge University Press; 1983

[16] Gilligan C. Con voce di donna. Etica e Formazione della personalità. Feltrinelli Milano; 1991

[17] Campagna AF, Harter S. Moral judgements in sociopathic and normal children. Journal of Personality and Social Psychology. 1975;**31**:199-205

[18] Blasi A. Bridging moral cognition and moral action: a critical review of the literature. Psychological Bulletin. 1980;**88**:1-45

[19] Blair RJR. A cognitive developmental approach to morality: Investigating the psychopath. Cognition. 1995;**57**:1-29

[20] Colby A, Kohiberg L. The Measurement of Moral Judgment. New York: Cambridge University Press; 1987

[21] Fodor EM. Delinquency and susceptibility of social influence among adolescents as a function of moral development. Journal of Social Psychology. 1972;**86**:257-260

[22] Hudgins W, Prentice NM. Moral judgment in delinquent and non delinquent adolescents and their mothers. Journal of Abnormal Psychology. 1973;**82**:145-152

[23] Jurkovic GJ, Prentice PM. Relation of moral and cognitive development to dimensions of juvenile delinquency. Journal of Abnormal Psychology. 1977;**86**:414-420

[24] Glenn AL, Raine A. Psicopatia. Introduzione alle scoperte biologiche e implicazioni. Giovanni Fioritti Roma; 2016

[25] Porges EG, Docety S. Violence as a source of pleasure or displeasure is associated with specific functional connectivity with the nucleus accumbens. Frontiers in Human Neuroscience. 2013;**7**:447

[26] Bowlby J. Attaccamento e perdita. Boringhieri Torino; 1999

[27] Anderson SM, Gedo PM. Relational trauma: Using play therapy to treat a disrupted attachment. Bulletin of the Menninger Clinic. 2013;**77**(3):250-268

[28] Schechter DS, Moser DA, Pointet VC, Aue T, Stenz L, Paoloni-Giacobino A, Adouan W, Manini A, Suardi F, Vital M, Sancho Rossignol A, Cordero MI, Rothenberg M, Ansermet F, Rusconi Serpa S, Dayer AG. The association of serotonin receptor 3A methylation with maternal violence exposure, neural activity, and child aggression. Behavioural Brain Research. 2016. **325**(Pt B): 268-277

[29] Meloy JR. The Psychopathic Mind: Origins, Dynamics, and Treatment. Jason Aronson Inc NY; 2002

[30] Cleckley H. The Mask of Sanity. St. Louis, MO: Mosby; 1941

[31] Cleckley H. The Mask of Sanity. 5th ed. St. Louis, MO: Mosby; 1976

[32] Hare RD. Diagnosis of antisocial personality disorder in two prison populations. American Journal of Psychiatry. 1983;**140**:887-890

[33] Hare RD. Hare Psychopathy Checklist Revised (PCL-R): Technical Manual. North Tonawanda, NY: Multi-Health Systems; 2003

[34] Neumann CS, Hare RD, Newman JP. The super-ordinate nature of the Psychopathy Checklist. Revised. Journal of Personality Disorders. 2007;**21**:102-117

[35] Caretti V, Schimmetti A. Trauma evolutivo e personalità psicopatica. XII Congresso Naz. Della Sezione Dinamica e Clinica. Torino: Associazione Italiana Psicologia; 2010. pp. 50-51

[36] Caretti V, Schimmetti A. Disturbed individuals or disturbing realities? Childood interpersonal trauma, violent attachment and psychopathy. In: 11th European Conference and Traumatic Stress; 2009; p. 49

[37] Hare RD. Without Conscience: The Disturbing World of Psychopaths Among is. New York: Pocket Books; 1993

[38] Millon T, Davis R. Disorders of Personality DSM IV and Beyond. Wiley Ed. New York; 1996

[39] Rosenfeld B, Pivovarova E. Test psicologici nella valutazione del rischio di violenza. In: Simon RI, Tardiff K, editors. Valutazione e gestione della violenza. Springer Milano; 2014

[40] Large M, Nielssen O. The limitations and future of violence risk assessment. World Psychiatry. 2017;**16**(1):25-26

[41] American Psychiatric Association. Diagnostic and Statistical Manual of Mental Disorders. Washington, DC: Author; 1952

[42] American Psychiatric Association. Diagnostic and Statistical Manual of Mental Disorders. 2nd ed. Washington, DC: Author; 1968

[43] American Psychiatric Association. Diagnostic and Statistical Manual of Mental Disorders. 3rd ed. Washington, DC: Author; 1980

[44] Spitzer RL, Williams JBW, Skodol AE. DSM-III: The major achievements and an overview. American Journal of Psychiatry. 1980;**137**:151-164

[45] Feighner JP, Robins E, Guze SB, Woodruff RA, Winokur G, Muñoz R. Diagnostic criteria for use in psychiatric research. Archives of General Psychiatry. 1972;**26**:57-63

[46] Robins LN. Deviant Children Grown Up. Baltimore: Williams & Wilkins; 1966

[47] American Psychiatric Association. Diagnostic and Statistical Manual of Mental Disorders. 3rd ed.rev. Washington, DC: Author; 1987

[48] Crego C, Widiger TA. Psychopathy and the DSM. Journal of Personality Disorders. 2015;**83**(6):665-677

[49] Widiger TA, Frances AJ, Spitzer RL, Williams JBW. The DSM-III-R personality disorders: An overview. American Journal of Psychiatry. 1988;**145**:786-795

[50] American Psychiatric Association. Diagnostic and Statistical Manual of Mental Disorders. 4th ed., text rev.. Washington, DC: Author; 1994

[51] American Psychiatric Association. Diagnostic and Statistical Manual of Mental Disorders, Fifth Edition (DSM-5). Arlington: American Psychiatric Association; 2013

[52] Patrick CJ, editor. Handbook of Psychopathy. New York: Guilford Press; 2006

[53] Patrick CJ, Fowles DC, Krueger RF. Triarchic conceptualization of psychopathy: Developmental origins of disinhibition, boldness, and meanness. Development and Psychopathology. 2009;**21**:913-938

[54] Lilienfeld SO, Widows MR. Psychopathic Personality Inventory-Revised professional manual. Lutz, FL: Psychological Assessment Resources; 2005

[55] Lynam DR, Gaughan E, Miller JD, Miller D, Mullins-Sweat S, Widiger TA. Assessing the basic traits associated with psychopathy: Development and validation of the Elemental Psychopathy Assessment. Psychological Assessment. 2011;**23**:108-124

[56] Skeem JL, Cooke DJ. Is criminal behavior a central component of psychopathy? Conceptual directions for resolving the debate. Psychological Assessment. 2010;**22**:433-445

[57] Lilienfeld SO, Patrick CJ, Benning SD, Berg J, Sellbom M, Edens JF. The role of fearless dominance in psychopathy: Confusions, controversies, and clarifications. Personality Disorders: Theory, Research, and Treatment. 2012;**3**:327-340

[58] Lamm C, Majdandžić J. The role of shared neural activations, mirror neurons, and morality in empathy—A critical comment. Neuroscience Research. 2015;**90**:15-24

[59] Baird AD, Scheffer IE, Wilson SJ. Mirror neuron system involvement in empathy: A critical look at the evidence. Society for Neuroscience. 2011;**6**(4):327-335

[60] Dutton K, McNab A. The Good Psychopath's Guide to Success. ; Bantam Press London; 2014

[61] Lilienfeld S, Latzman RD, Smith SF, Dutton K. Correlate of psychopathic personality traits in everyday life: Results from a large community survey. Frontiers in Psychology. 2014;**5**:740

[62] Lorettu L. Le reazioni emotive al paziente violento: implicazioni diagnostiche e terapeutiche. CSE, Torino; 2000

Chapter 2

Development of Psychopathy from Childhood

Merve Cikili Uytun

Additional information is available at the end of the chapter

http://dx.doi.org/10.5772/intechopen.70119

Abstract

Serious conduct problems are a serious mental health and public policy concern. Such conduct problems are highly related to criminal behavior and are associated with a host of other social, emotional, and academic problems. In addition, serious conduct problems in childhood predict later impairments in the domains of mental health, legal, educational, social, occupational, and physical health. In the past two decades, a significant body of research has emerged refining how the key features associated with psychopathy may be expressed in children and adolescents. These researches have focused largely on the presence of callous-unemotional traits, which correspond closely to the affective dimension of psychopathy—core to the construct in adult samples. Several reviews have focused on important theoretical questions related to how best to identify psychopathy in children and adolescents but do not directly address their importance for understanding, classifying, and treating youths with severe conduct problems. So, in the forefront of these studies, I aimed to review the development of psychopathy from childhood. In this chapter, topics related to psychopathy, such as diagnosis and nosology, epidemiologic studies, etiologic factors, assessment, diagnostic interviews, comorbid disorders and longitudinal outcome, treatment modalities, and treatment outcome in samples of children and adolescents, were included.

Keywords: child, adolescent, psychopathy, conduct, development

1. Introduction

Psychopathy is defined as complex disorder of personality conceptualized by a constellation of behavioral attributes and personality traits centered on one of three main dimensions: (a) an impulsive/antisocial lifestyle, (b) callous, arrogant, and deceitful interpersonal behavior, or (c) deficient affective responses [1].

It has strong associations with criminality and recidivism [2], and those with high levels of psychopathy are likely to relate in both reactive and premeditated aggression and to demonstrate little remorse for their actions [3].

Conduct disorder, antisocial personality disorder, and psychopathy are known as developmental disorders and the terms can be used interchangeably sometimes. However, there are significant differences between them and related factors [4]. Conduct disorder and antisocial personality disorder primarily focus on behavioral problems, but differently, Hare's psychopathy describe is emphasized that deficits in affective and interpersonal functioning [3]. However, people with these traits exhibit a more severe, violent, and chronic pattern of antisocial behavior [5, 6]. Understanding the construct of psychopathy is important to the legal system, to the mental health system, and for research attempting to explain the causes of antisocial and aggressive behavior. Importantly, research has shown that adults with psychopathic traits often have long histories of antisocial behavior that often extend well into childhood [7].

As a result, there have been numerous attempts to define developmental precursors to psychopathy. In this chapter, we reviewed the development of psychopathy from childhood and related issues in children and adolescents.

2. Diagnosis and nosology

For many years, the construct of psychopathy has had an important role in understanding antisocial behavior and criminality in adults, and the adult psychopathy literature provides the foundation for the youth psychopathy construct [8].

Regardless of disagreement and debate concerning the structure and measurement of the psychopathy construct theories in the adult literature, interest has grown in examining psychopathic traits in youth. First, the strong associations between psychopathy factors and antisocial behavior and violence in the adult literature have prompted interest in whether conduct problems, aggression, and violence in some youth might be explained by similar personality correlates [9]. Second, Lynam has proposed that, to prevent the serious negative outcomes associated with psychopathy, the early identification of psychopathic traits is essential because (a) attempts to treat psychopathy in adulthood have proven to be quite unsuccessful [10, 11]; and (b) evidence suggests that psychopathic individuals have antisocial and criminal histories that begin prior to adulthood [8].

Before the recent increased interest in psychopathic traits in youth, attempts already have been made to improve the psychopathy construct to juveniles. The DSM-III was categorized children with conduct disorder (CD) who were "socialized" or "undersocialized." The undersocialized type was characterized by a failure to experience normal degrees of affection, empathy, or interpersonal bonds; a lack of peer relationships; egocentrism; manipulation; callous behavior; and a lack of guilt type, and it was clearly connected to the adult psychopathic personality. In contrast, "the socialized type of CD was characterized by behaviors that were similar to those currently associated with the deviant lifestyle factor." Within this system, youth were also categorized as aggressive/nonaggressive [12].

Research using these DSM-III categories revealed that undersocialized aggressive children were more likely to have continued CD into adulthood and generally poorer developmental outcomes [13, 14].

However, DSM-III listed only one symptom specific to the "affective and interpersonal dimensions of psychopathy (i.e., does not 'apparently feel guilt or remorse when such a reaction is appropriate not just when caught or in difficulty'). The other four symptoms focused on indicators of social attachment (e.g., does not have 'one or more peer group friendships that have lasted over 6 months'), which have not proven to be highly indicative of the construct of psychopathy in samples of children and adolescents" [15].

As a result of these definitional problems, the undersocialized distinction was not continued in later editions of the DSM. In the next version of the DSM (DSM-III-R; American Psychiatric Association [16]), the CD subtyping criteria were revised to focus on more easily measured behavioral criteria [16]. This change moved the CD subtyping criteria farther from a focus on interpersonal and affective factors that were closely tied to adult psychopathy [17]. As a result of this change, conceptualizations about the development of child behavior problems were also changed; researches in the conduct problems literature became increasingly focused on specific antisocial behaviors in children and less focused on psychological dimensions related to antisocial behavior [18, 19].

Some models were suggested for subtyping of aggression and psychopathy in children and adolescent. First, childhood onset conduct disorder and Attention Deficit and Hyperactivity Disorder (ADHD) may be precursors for psychopathy in children and adolescents. In support of this approach, there have been several reviews indicating that children with both types of problems show a more severe and aggressive pattern of antisocial behavior than children with conduct problems alone [20, 21]. But all of these patients are not related at higher risk for antisocial and criminal outcomes in adulthood. Another subtyping method for these children that two forms of aggression can be identified in samples of children or adolescents with conduct problems [22, 23]. Reactive aggression is characterized by impulsive-defensive responses to a perceived provocation or threat and is usually accompanied by a display of intense physiological reactivity [24, 25]. However, proactive or instrumental aggression is usually intended and it is not associated with provocation [22, 24]. The second group is similar to adult offenders with psychopathic traits who have been shown to be more aggressive [26, 27].

However, in the past two decades, a significant body of research has emerged refining how the key features associated with psychopathy may be expressed in children and adolescents [15, 28]. These conceptualizations have focused largely on the "presence of callous-unemotional (CU) traits (e.g., lack of empathy and guilt, failure to put for the effort on important tasks, shallow and deficient emotions), which correspond closely to the affective dimension of psychopathy—core to the construct in adult samples" [29]. An increased literature has accumulated regarding psychological and behavioral differences between impulsive conduct-disordered (high I/CP) children exhibiting low versus high levels of CU tendencies [30–32]. The studies with nonclinic control children, high CU clinic-referred youth, and high I/CP children with low levels of CU features are prone to reactive aggression, but not proactive aggression. In addition, compared with control group, high CU conduct-problem children exhibit high levels of proactive as well as reactive aggression. Relatedly, there is evidence that the presence of CU traits prospectively predicts later incidence of aggression and violence over and above I/CP tendencies [33].

As a result of these studies, the most recent revision of the Diagnostic and Statistical Manual of Mental Disorders (American Psychiatric Association [34]) has integrated these changes into the diagnostic criteria for conduct disorder.

The DSM-5 criteria for conduct disorder were presented below:

A. Repetitive and persistent pattern of behavior in which the basic rights of others or major age-appropriate societal norms or rules are violated, as manifested by the presence of at least three of the following 15 criteria in the past 12 months from any of the categories below, with at least one criterion present in the past 6 months:

Aggression to people and animals

1. Often bullies, threatens, or intimidates others.

2. Often initiates physical fights.

3. Has used a weapon that can cause serious physical harm to others (e.g., a bat, brick, broken bottle, knife, gun).

4. Has been physically cruel to people.

5. Has been physically cruel to animals.

6. Has stolen while confronting a victim (e.g., mugging, purse snatching, extortion, armed robbery).

7. Has forced someone into sexual activity.

Destruction of property

8. Has deliberately engaged in fire setting with the intention of causing serious damage.

9. Has deliberately destroyed others' property (other than by fire setting).

Deceitfulness or theft

10. Has broken into someone else's house, building, or car.

11. Often lies to obtain goods or favors or to avoid obligations (i.e., "cons" others).

12. Has stolen items of nontrivial value without confronting a victim (e.g., shoplifting, but without breaking and entering; forgery).

Serious violations of rules

13. Often stays out at night despite parental prohibitions, beginning before age 13 years.

14. Has run away from home overnight at least twice while living in the parental or parental surrogate home, or once without returning for a lengthy period.

15. Is often truant from school, beginning before age 13 years.

B. The disturbance in behavior causes clinically significant impairment in social, academic, or occupational functioning.

C. If the individual is 18 years or older, criteria are not met for antisocial personality disorder.

Specify whether:

Childhood-onset type: Individuals show at least one symptom characteristic of conduct disorder prior to age 10 years.

Adolescent-onset type: Individuals show no symptom characteristic of conduct disorder prior to age 10 years.

Unspecified onset: Criteria for a diagnosis of conduct disorder are met, but there is not enough information available to determine whether the onset of the first symptom was before or after age 10 years.

Specify if:

With limited prosocial emotions: To qualify for this specifier, an individual must have displayed at least two of the following characteristics persistently over at least 12 months and in multiple relationships and settings. These characteristics reflect the individual's typical pattern of interpersonal and emotional functioning over this period and not just occasional occurrences in some situations. Thus, to assess the criteria for the specifier, multiple information sources are necessary. In addition to the individual's self-report, it is necessary to consider reports by others who have known the individual for extended periods of time (e.g., parents, teachers, co-workers, extended family members, peers).

Lack of remorse or guilt: Does not feel bad or guilty when he or she does something wrong (exclude remorse when expressed only when caught and/or facing punishment). The individual shows a general lack of concern about the negative consequences of his or her actions. For example, the individual is not remorseful after hurting someone or does not care about the consequences of breaking rules.

Callous—lack of empathy: Disregards and is unconcerned about the feelings of others. The individual is described as cold and uncaring. The person appears more concerned about the effects of his or her actions on himself or herself, rather than their effects on others, even when they result in substantial harm to others.

Unconcerned about performance: Does not show concern about poor/problematic performance at school, at work, or in other important activities. The individual does not put forth the effort necessary to perform well, even when expectations are clear, and typically blame others for his or her poor performance.

Shallow or deficient affect: Does not express feelings or show emotions to others, except in ways that seem shallow, insincere, or superficial (e.g., actions contradict the emotion displayed; can turn emotions "on" or "off" quickly) or when emotional expressions are used for gain (e.g., emotions displayed to manipulate or intimidate others).

Specify current severity:

Mild: Few, if any, conduct problems in excess of those required to make the diagnosis are present, and conduct problems cause relatively minor harm to others (e.g., lying, truancy, staying out after dark without permission, other rule breaking).

Moderate: The number of conduct problems and the effect on others intermediate between those specified in "mild" and those in "severe" (e.g., stealing without confronting a victim, vandalism).

Severe: Many conduct problems in excess of those required to make the diagnosis are present, or conduct problems cause considerable harm to others (e.g., forced sex, physical cruelty, use of a weapon, stealing while confronting a victim, breaking and entering) [34].

We concluded that all of studies about this issue were implicated that CU traits are most studied predictors for psychopathy in children and adolescents.

3. Epidemiology

Children with conduct problems (CP), commonly identified as either having oppositional defiant disorder (ODD) or conduct disorder (CD), comprise about 5–10% of youth aged 8–16 years [35]. Prevalence of CP is even higher in preschool populations ranging from 7 to 25% [36]. In a study, the prevalence for psychopathy in young offender sample was 21.5% [37], and the prevalence rate found for adult psychopathy ranges from approximately 15–30% [38]. In a population of adolescents involved with criminal or psychiatric services, using a Psychopathy Checklist—Youth Version (PCL–YV) cut-off score of >30 psychopathy, Forth and Burke found rates of 3.5% in young people in community care, 12% in those on probation, and 28.3% in those incarcerated [39]. Brandt et al. using PCL–YV cut-off score of >28 reported a prevalence of 37% in incarcerated youths [40].

No epidemiological data exist that directly quantify the prevalence rates of psychopathy across the population; however, people have used data from forensic and clinical samples to estimate that approximately 0.75–1% of the population may be psychopaths. A similar percentage of children present with both severe antisocial behavior and CU features. It is estimated that there are more males than females presenting with these traits, although the gender ratio is unclear [41].

4. Etiology

4.1. Genetic factors

Several studies examined the heritability of CU traits, and these studies provided estimates of the amount of variation in CU traits accounted for by genetic effects ranging from 42 to 68% [42–45]. Additionally, although a large proportion of the correlation between CU traits and conduct problems has been reported to be due to shared genetic effects, studies have consistently found unique genetic influences to both constructs as well supporting at least partially distinct etiological underpinnings [44, 46–48]. In a study of 7-year-old twins, the genetic influences on childhood-onset conduct problems were teacher-reported CU traits (81%) higher than normal group (30%) [49]. The research team also found that the level of genetic influence on conduct problems in those with increased levels of CU traits was not related to the severity of conduct problems and it was not related to ADHD symptoms when the children were 9 years of age [50].

Specifically, one twin study in a sample of boys aged 10–13 reported that left posterior cingulate and right dorsal anterior cingulate gray matter concentrations showed significant heritability (0.46 and 0.37) and that common genes explained the phenotypic relationship between these regions and psychopathic traits and these data suggest that the genetic contribution to CU traits might manifest through an impact on anterior and posterior cingulate cortex development [51].

Several studies have investigated potential genetic polymorphisms associated with CU traits. Especially, Viding et al. documented several potential autosomal single-nucleotide polymorphisms that could play a role in the development of CU traits [52]. Furthermore, Hirata et al. explored the role of COMT gene variants in child aggression and in CU traits and they reported CU traits among children and adolescents were associated with two catechol O-methyltransferase (COMT) polymorphisms [53]. COMT is an enzyme that metabolizes catecholamines including dopamine and norepinephrine, and its activity is mainly located in the frontal areas of the brain, including regions important in regulating aggressive behavior. Male mice lacking COMT displayed increased aggression [54]. Fowler et al. also found evidence to suggest that COMT polymorphisms may be related to CU traits. Additionally, they explored also MAO-A and 5-HTT genes among adolescents (ages 12–19) with childhood ADHD, they demonstrated that the high activity COMT Val/Val genotype, a low activity monoamine oxidase-a receptor (MAO-A) allele, and who were homozygous for the low activity serotonin transporter (5-HTT) allele significantly higher associated with CU traits [55]. In another study of 162 children and adolescents (ages 6–16), CU traits were associated with two polymorphisms on the oxytocin receptor (OSTR) gene [56]. Finally, in a recent study, Hirata et al. explore the role of prolactin and prolactin receptor gene (PRLR) variants in child aggression and CU traits. They found that one of the three single-nucleotide polymorphisms (SNPs) of the PRLR gene (rs187490) was significantly associated with CU traits and participants who carrying the GG genotype having higher CU scores than A-allele carriers [57].

Another promising candidate is FKBP5, which codes for a protein, FK506 binding protein, and regulates the affinity of the glucocorticoid receptor for cortisol [58]. The most prominent polymorphism in this gene (rs1360780) has been linked to increased aggression. Specifically, an interaction effect of FKBP5 diplotypes and childhood trauma was found on lifetime aggressive behavior in 411 male prisoners; carriers of the diplotype linked to increased FKBP5 expression were found to exhibit increased aggression and violent behavior in jail following childhood abuse [59]. This finding has been replicated on a brain imaging by two studies showing that FKBP5 variants interacted with childhood adversity to predict threat-induced activity in the amygdala [60, 61].

A small number of candidate genes (e.g., COMT, MAOA, OSTR, PRLR) are associated with CU traits across independent studies; however, failures to replicate also exist. Studies of gene-environment interplay show that CU traits genetic predispositions also contribute to selection into higher risk environments and that environmental factors can alter the differentially methylated CU trait candidate genes. The field's understanding of CU traits etiology will benefit from larger, adequately powered studies in gene identification efforts; the incorporation of polygenic approaches in gene-environment interplay studies; attention to the mechanisms of risk from genes to brain to behavior; and the use of genetically informative data to test quasi-causal hypotheses about purported risk factors.

In the future, genetic findings can predict whether aggression will occur in children and it will persist into adulthood, and it may be possible to provide preventive interventions or more targeted treatments for those at high risk. Overall, with further genetic researches may lead to new avenues of risk prediction, prevention, and treatment of aggressive behaviors.

4.2. Temperament and personality

In the researches of this area, the most consistent finding is that CU traits are associated with lower levels of fear and lower levels of anxiety (or neuroticism) [62], although, as a group children with conduct problems showed higher levels of trait anxiety (perhaps secondary to the stressors they experience as a result of their maladaptive behaviors) [63].

Fearlessness is central to developmental models of psychopathy and increasing risk for callous-unemotional behaviors [64]. In recent study, it was shown that fearless temperament at age 2 predicted both CU traits and conduct problems at age 13 [65].

Another temperament dimension central to psychopathy is low affiliative behavior, operationalized as low interpersonal warmth or affection. Although direct prospective links from low affiliative behavior have not been tested, recent studies suggest that callous-unemotional behaviors are related to lower quality of positive affective parent-child interactions, including lower eye contact, warmth, [66, 67] and empathy [68].

Additionally, narcissistic traits have been found positively associated with CU traits [69–71].

In summary, the studies demonstrate that although fearlessness and low affiliative behavior are passed from mother to child and that increasing risk for callous-unemotional behaviors, highly positive parenting can buffer risk.

4.3. Neurobiological factors

Functional abnormalities of amygdala are the most consistent findings in psychopathic-like adolescents. Adolescents with conduct problems and callous-unemotional traits show less amygdala responsiveness to fearful faces (but not other emotional expressions) compared to healthy controls [72–75] and compared to children with conduct problems but low CU traits [76]. Functional imaging studies of children and adolescents have also found youths with both conduct problems and either psychopathic traits exhibit lower right amygdala activity during an affective theory of mind task [77].

Another imaging study showed that youths with CD or ODD and high levels of psychopathic traits showed disruptions in amygdala-prefrontal functional connectivity [78]. The same research group reported that youths with both conduct problems (aged 10–17 years) and elevated CU traits demonstrated increased activity bilaterally in the medial frontal gyri and abnormal activity within the ventromedial prefrontal cortex during punished reversal errors compared to normal controls. This shows that psychopathic traits are associated with abnormal processing of reinforcement information [79].

In contrast to functional imaging, there have been null findings regarding the structural integrity of the amygdala in children with CU traits [80, 81]. Wallace et al. found reduced amygdala volumes in children with CD but they noted that CU traits were not effective on this volume. Also, in another study found that "reduced amygdala gray matter volume in adolescents with CD, but no significant differences associated with CU traits" [82]. One structural imaging study reported that, compared to normal developing boys, boys with both conduct problems and elevated CU traits showed increased gray matter concentration in the medial orbitofrontal and anterior cingulate cortex, in addition to increased gray matter volume and concentration in the temporal lobes bilaterally [81]. Additionally, "this finding is consistent with the findings of the twin study reported previously showing that common genes seemed to explain the association between right dorsal anterior cingulate gray matter concentrations and psychopathic traits" [51]. In the recent study, it were explored that longitudinal data spanning an average of 22 years to comprehensively examine whether adult male subjects with low amygdala volume have a longstanding developmental history of aggression and psychopathic features that persist into the future. They found that men with lower amygdala volume associated with higher levels of aggressive behavior and psychopathic traits from childhood. It was found that in adolescence and young adulthood, lower amygdala volume was also associated with proactive aggression. More importantly, "this is the first study to demonstrate that adult men with lower amygdala volume were at increased risk for exhibiting future aggression, violence, and psychopathic traits, even after controlling for earlier levels of these features and several potential confounds" [83].

Prefrontal cortex and its role in psychopathy in children and adolescents is increasing in the researchs, in the literature, there is a few studies about structural MRI. Two studies found that psychopathic adolescents who were incarcerated had decreased gray matter volumes in the orbitofrontal cortex [84, 85]. In contrast, De Brito et al. found increased gray matter concentration in the medial orbitofrontal cortex and anterior cingulate cortex of boys with elevated CU traits. This finding led to note that "normal cortical maturation involves gray matter loss, and consequently their finding of increased gray matter in their juveniles may reflect a delay in prefrontal maturation" [81]. Finger et al. compared youth with disruptive behavior disorders (DBD) to healthy controls and showed "hypoactivity in the orbitofrontal cortex in response to early stimulus-reinforcement exposure and rewards." The psychopathic adolescents demonstrated reduced neural activity when the task was related to stimuli-reinforcement associations, when they completed the task correctly, and when they were rewarded [86].

White et al. investigated the relationship between a large cavum septum pellucidum (CSP) and symptom severity in disruptive behavior disorders (DBD; conduct disorder and oppositional defiant disorder). They observed that individuals with a large CSP have a higher risk for aggressive behavior, psychopathic traits, and being diagnosed ODD/CD. However, it should be noted that the presence of a large CSP was not associated with a more severe form of DBD (CD vs. ODD) [87].

Resting state fMRI (rs-fMRI) studies are also limited in this area. We found three rs-fMRI studies with CD: firstly Zhou et al. found that the CD participants showed decreased the amplitude of low-frequency fluctuations (ALFF) in the bilateral amygdala/parahippocampus, right lingual gyrus, left cuneus, and right insula and greater ALFF was showed in the right fusiform gyrus and right thalamus in the CD group compared to the TD group [88]. The other study implicated that adolescents with CD showed decreased functional connectivity within the bilateral PCC, bilateral precuneus, and right superior temporal gyrus relative to TD group. It could be speculated that CD is associated with decreased functional connectivity within the default mode network (DMN) and between the DMN and other regions [89, 90]. Cikili-Uytun et al. found that increased DMN activity in ADHD+CD group compared to ADHD and in the ADHD group compared to controls in several DMN regions. This result is consistent with rs-fMRI studies, which showed that the increased DMN with ADHD but different from the study which showed decreased DMN activity with CD adolescents [91]. Increased activity in the DMN was present in some previous studies, and this study is consistent with the hypothesis that ADHD individuals may have increased disturbances during task performance and that reflect faulty deactivation of the DMN [92]. They speculated that this hypothesis is also could be reason for CD. But all of inthese resting state studies, CU traits did not differ from in the conduct disorder criteria.

With some exceptions, the majority of studies to date have demonstrated reduced function, volume, and connectivity in the frontal cortex and the amygdala in psychopathic adults and adolescents; two brain areas strongly implicated in prosocial behavior and decision making. Amygdala plays role in different functions such as fear of punishment, or aversion to causing fear/pain and impaired amygdala functioning and structure would lead to disturbances in antisocial children and adolescents. The prefrontal cortex is implicated in a number of functions such as executive functioning, impulse control, moral decision-making, reward and punishment processing, behavioral inhibition, and planning for the future, and if it was impaired, it would have significant influence on tendency toward antisocial behavior.

Although more imaging studies are needed, especially comparing children and adolescents with conduct problems with and without elevated levels of CU traits, these studies are implicated that the neurological markers for some of the emotional and cognitive characteristics of children and adolescents with severe conduct problems and elevated CU traits [93].

4.4. Cognitive factors

One consistent finding related to cognitive studies is that CU traits are associated with abnormalities in the processing of punishment cues. Specifically, CU traits have been associated with an insensitivity to punishment cues and the youth has to respond to an increasing ratio of punished to rewarded responses [94, 95]. Blair et al. explored different punishment schedules, youths with behavior problems and high levels of psychopathic traits have been reported as responding more poorly to gradual punishment compared to youths with behavior problems but normative levels of psychopathic traits. In addition, boys with elevated CU traits were less sensitive to potential punishment when compared to boys with normative levels of CU traits [96]. Blair et al. also found children with psychopathic tendencies made significantly more errors when processing fearful expressions than the comparison group, and they were also significantly less sensitive to sad expressions than the comparison group, as indicated by increased response stage to sadness [97].

Dadds et al. explored whether children with high CU traits are in fact callous and unemotional across all situations or whether they demonstrate emotional responsiveness and emotion regulation strategies in response to complex fear and attachment-related stimuli. They found that children in the high CU traits group expressed more happiness in the fear scene than the low-CU and healthy children. In the attachment scenario, high CU children expressed similar higher emotional responses and emotion regulation strategies than low CU children and control children. The results support the idea that high CU children may have the potential for emotional responsiveness to complex emotional stimuli in attachment contexts [98].

Also, several studies reported that children and adolescents with severe conduct problems and elevated CU traits show deviant social responses that include viewing aggression as a more acceptable means for obtaining goals, blaming others for their misbehavior, and emphasizing the importance of dominance and revenge in social conflicts [99–102].

Deficits in affective empathy (i.e., experiencing negative emotions due to the harm caused to others) were consistently reported that associated with CU traits [102–104], and this association remains significant after controlling for level of impulsivity and conduct problems [100] and level of aggression [105]. However, the association between CU traits and deficits in cognitive empathy (i.e., the ability to take the perspective of others) has been reported in some studies [102, 106, 107].

In the children and adolescents, who have conduct problems and CU traits, intelligence was examined in four clusters. They found that "the conduct problems—only cluster had a lower average full scale intelligence score compared to the cluster of children with both conduct problems and CU traits and the cluster with low conduct problems and low CU traits" [108]. Loney et al. replicated these results in a sample of 117 clinic-referred children (6–13 years old) and found that, compared to a clinical control group, children with conduct problems demonstrated a verbal intelligence deficit only in the absence of CU traits [109].

Some studies reported that adolescents with both conduct problems and elevated levels of CU traits were less impaired in their verbal abilities [109, 110], were less likely to show a hostile attribution bias [95], and showed greater flexibility in developing solutions in social problem-solving tasks [111] than other adolescents with conduct problems. However, such evidence for less impaired cognitive abilities in youths with elevated CU traits has not been found in all studies [112, 113] and requires further testing.

In summary, the available research strongly suggests that children and adolescents with conduct problems and higher levels of CU traits differ from other youths with conduct problems by showing abnormalities in the processing of punishment cues, by endorsing more deviant social goals, and by showing deficits in affective empathy. In contrast, deficits in cognitive empathy and cognitive perspective taking have not been as consistently documented with elevated levels of CU traits in children and adolescents.

4.5. Parenting and environmental factors

The most consistent finding from these studies is that parenting factors tend to have different associations with conduct problems depending on whether it is accompanied by high levels of CU traits. Many studies that have tested the moderating role of CU traits in the association between parenting and serious conduct problems focus on harsh discipline, lack of parental warmth, or inconsistency in parenting practices. Studies examining these aspects of negative parenting practices are more strongly related to conduct problems in those low on CU traits. Specifically, harsh, inconsistent, and coercive discipline has consistently been shown to be more highly associated with conduct problems in youths with normative levels of CU traits [114–116]. In the studies, it is found that chronically elevated levels of callousness have been longitudinally related to harsh parenting in children aged 2–4 years [117], as well as poor parent-child communication among male adolescents with symptoms of ODD/CD [118]. Longitudinal studies have found evidence that positive parenting relates to lower rates of externalizing problems later in childhood for youth with elevated levels of CU traits [119, 120]. Additionally, in some studies, low warmth as another factor in parenting appears to be more highly associated with conduct problems in youths with elevated CU traits [116, 121].

Also several studies have investigated associations between psychopathic traits and attachment style; especially dismissive attachment and disorganized attachment style were found related with psychopathic traits [116, 122]. Dadds et al. explored the problems related to attachment and they reported that children with high levels of CU traits made less eye contact with their parents in both free play and in "emotional talk" situations, different from ADHD and conduct problems [123].

In the literature, it is known that the prevalence of reported physical, emotional, and sexual abuse were higher in the delinquent youth than control group [124–126]. Krischer and Sevecke showed that relationships between physical traumatization and the CU traits could be confirmed among criminal boys, but not among delinquent girls. However, they found that in girls, other family-related variables, such as nonparental living arrangements, seemed to be more influential in developing the psychopathy syndrome than traumatization [127].

Very minimal research has been conducted on the peer groups of children with elevated levels of CU traits. In one of the few studies, Muñoz et al. reported that, although adolescents with high levels of CU traits had as many friends as other adolescents, the friendships were less stable and were viewed as more controversial [128]. Another study showed that peer victimization at age 10 predicted CU traits at age 13 in children who scored high on a measure of irritability [129]. One consistent finding on the peer groups of children and adolescents with high levels of CU traits is often associate with delinquent and antisocial peers, and this level of deviant friendship seems to be higher than in children and adolescents with conduct problems but without CU traits [118, 130, 131].

In summary, it can be made based on the available research on parenting practices is that harsh and coercive parenting appears to have stronger associations with conduct problems in those without significant levels of CU traits. However, a few studies have suggested that warm parenting may be directly related negatively to CU traits or to the conduct problems displayed by children and adolescents with elevated CU traits. Furthermore, there may be some subgroups of children and adolescents with elevated CU traits whose problems are more likely to have developed as a result of harsh and abusive parenting.

Also, although it is clear that adolescents with CU traits tend to associate with deviant and antisocial peers, data are limited about the peer relationships of youths with higher CU traits.

4.6. Other biological factors

Most of the studies show that some psychophysiological factors correlates to CU traits in children and adolescents with nonnormative levels of CU traits. Two studies were found that youths with both CD and higher CU traits showed a lower changing of heart rate to emotionally reminiscent films compared to youths with CD but without CU traits [132, 133]. In addition, it was demonstrated that when anticipating aversive stimuli, skin conductance reactivity reduced in adolescents with psychopathic traits compared to controls [134, 135]. Additionally, CU traits were negatively related to skin conductance reactivity when responding to peer provocation in a sample of detained adolescent boys [136]. Finally, children with CU traits have shown blunted cortisol reactivity to experimentally induced stress [137].

Such studies are very limited and should replicate the current findings; it would provide more definitive support for the proposed etiological links between these biological factors and psychopathy.

In **Table 1**, genetic, neurobiological, and other biological factors were summarized.

Study	Sample	Results
Viding et al. [49]	N =7374; age =7; population-based community sample	Conduct problems in children high on CU traits showed stronger genetic influence than those low on CU traits
Viding et al. [50]	N =3730; age =9; population-based community sample	Conduct problems in children high on CU traits showed stronger genetic influence than those low on CU traits, even controlling for the presence of ADHD symptoms
Bezdjian et al. [42]	N = 1219; age =9–10; community sample	Significant genetic influences on psychopathic traits were found for both boys and girls
Rijsdijk et al. [51]	N = 123; age = 10–13; male; community sample	Left posterior cingulate and right dorsal anterior cingulate gray matter concentrations showed significant heritability, and common genes explained the phenotypic relationship between these regions and CU traits
Beitchman et al. [56]	N =162; age = 6–16; clinical sample	CU traits were associated with two polymorphisms on the oxytocin receptor (OXTR) gene alleles OXTR_rs237885 A allele and OXTR_rs2268493es A allele
Fowler et al. [55]	N = 147; age =12–19; clinical sample	Among adolescents with childhood ADHD, those possessing a low activity MAOA allele, those who were homozygous for the low activity 5HTT allele, and those with the high activity COMT Val/Val genotype demonstrated significantly higher CU traits even after controlling for CD
Hirata et al. [53]	N =144; age =6–16; clinic-referred sample	Within a sample of children and adolescents high on conduct problems, CU traits were associated with two COMT polymorphisms
Hirata et al. [57]	N = 123; age = 6–16 clinically referred sample	The one of the three SNPs of the PRLR gene was significantly associated with CU traits with participants carrying the GG genotype having higher CU scores than A-allele carriers

Study	Sample	Results
Marsh et al. [72]	N =36; age =10–17; community sample	Youths with elevated CU traits showed reduced amygdala activation while processing fearful expressions compared to youths with ADHD and normal controls
Jones et al. [73]	N =30; age =10–12; male, community twin sample	Boys with conduct problems and elevated CU traits demonstrated lower right amygdala activity in response to fearful faces
Finger et al. [79]	N =42; age =10–17; community sample	Youths with psychopathic traits demonstrated abnormal responses within the ventromedial prefrontal cortex during punished reversal errors
Sebastian et al. [77]	N =47; age 10–16; male community sample	CU traits demonstrated a negative association with activity in the right amygdala in response to affective Theory of Mind scenarios after controlling for conduct problems
White et al. [87]	N =20; age =11–17; community sample	While playing a social Exchange game, participants with higher levels of CU traits demonstrated a weaker relationship between increases in punishment of unfair offers and increased dorsal anterior cingulate cortex (dACC) and anterior insula activity
Finger et al. [78]	N =31; mean age =14.8, community sample	Youths with CD/ODD and high levels of psychopathic traits had disruptions in amygdala-prefrontal functional connectivity but no disruption in structural connections of the uncinate fasciculus or white matter tracts
Fairchild et al. [82]	N =42; age =14–20; mixed clinical and community sample	CU traits were positively associated with bilateral middle/superior orbitofrontal (OFC) volume controlling for lifetime history of CD and ADHD. Girls with CD and CU traits had reduced right anterior insula volume compared to girls with CD and normative levels of CU traits
De Brito et al. [81]	N =48; mean age = 11.7; male; community sample	Boys with conduct problems and elevated CU traits showed increased gray matter concentration in the medial orbitofrontal and anterior cingulate cortices in addition to increased gray matter volume and concentration in the temporal lobes bilaterally
White et al. [61]	N=59; mean age =14.90; community sample	Compared to controls, youths with ODD/CD had a larger CSP
Wallace et al. [80]	N=49; age=10–18; community sample	Youths with CD show reduced cortical thickness within superior temporal regions, some indications of reduced gyrification within ventromedial frontal cortex and reduced amygdala and striatum (putamen and pallidum) volumes.
Cope et al. [85]	N = 39; mean age = 17.6 years; incarcerated female adolescents	The regional gray matter volumes were negatively related to psychopathic traits in female youth offenders in limbic and paralimbic areas, including orbitofrontal cortex, parahippocampal cortex, temporal poles, and left hippocampus
Zhou et al. [88]	N=36; age = 15–17; forensic sample	Adolescents with CD showed significantly reduced functional connectivity within the bilateral posterior cingulate cortex (PCC), bilateral precuneus and right superior temporal gyrus relative to TD controls. CD is associated with reduced functional connectivity within the DMN and between the DMN and other regions
Zhou et al. [89]	N=36; age= 15–17; forensic sample	Compared with the TD participants, the CD participants showed lower ALFF in the bilateral amygdala/parahippocampus, right lingual gyrus, left cuneus, and right insula. Higher ALFF was observed in the right fusiform gyrus and right thalamus in the CD participants compared to the TD group

Study	Sample	Results
Uytun et al. [91]	N=30; age= 9–16; clinical sample	The findings revealed group differences between cingulate cortex and primary motor cortex; cingulate cortex and somatosensory association cortex; angular gyrus (AG) and dorsal posterior cingulate cortex, in these networks increased activity was observed in participants with ADHD+CD compared with the ADHD
Cheng et al. (2012)	N =28; age = 15–18; male; forensic sample	The offenders both low and high on psychopathic traits demonstrated higher pain thresholds. Youths high on psychopathic traits showed impairment in both early and late processing of empathy, evidenced by decreased frontal N120, central P3, and late positive potential (LPP)
Anastassiou-Hadjicharalambous and Warden [132]	N = 95; age =7–11; high-risk community sample and clinical sample	Youths with CD and elevated CU traits exhibited lower magnitude of heart rate change while watching an emotionally evocative film
De Wied et al. [133]	N =63; age =12–15; male; high-risk community sample	Resting RSA was significantly lower in youths with conduct problems and elevated CU traits compared to other conduct problem youths and age-matched normal controls. Youths with conduct problems and elevated CU traits also demonstrated less change in heart rate response to empathy inducing film clips involving sadness
Fung et al. [134]	N =130; age =16; male; community sample	Youths who scored high on psychopathic traits exhibited reduced skin conductance activity when anticipating and responding to aversive stimuli compared to control youths with normative levels of psychopathic traits
Isen et al. [135]	N =791; age =9–10; community sample	Boys with higher levels of psychopathic traits showed lower skin conductance reactivity (SCR) to unsignaled and nonaversive auditory stimuli There was no relationship between psychopathic traits and SCR hyporeactivity in girls
Kimonis et al. [136]	N =248; age=12–20; forensic sample	Higher levels of CU traits were associated with less empathy, less positive affect, and less skin conductance reactivity to provocations from peers
Stadler et al. [137]	N =36; age =8–14; male; clinical sample	Youths with ADHD, conduct problems, and high levels of CU traits exhibited blunted cortisol reactivity to experimentally induced stress compared to youths with normative levels of CU traits

Table 1. Genetic, neurobiological, and other biological etiological factors.

5. Assesment and diagnostic interviews

Several instruments that were specifically designed to assess psychopathic traits in children and adolescents are currently available [138].

5.1. Psychopathy checklist—youth version (PCL–YV)

The PCL–YV is a 20-item rating scale and the items are scored on the basis of information from a semistructured interview and file review. The PCL–YV has modified item descriptions but it was seen the nearly same on the adult measure. These modifications are intended to take into consideration adolescent life experiences with an increased emphasis on peer, family, and school adjustment. The PCL–YV is scored on a 3-point scale in which 0 indicates the characteristic is consistently absent, 1 indicates the characteristic is inconsistently present, and 2 indicates the characteristic is consistently present [139].

5.2. Antisocial process screening device (APSD)

The APSD is a 20-item self-report measure and it was designed to assess traits associated with the construct of psychopathy similar the Psychopathy Checklist—Revised (PCL–R; Hare, 1991). The APSD was originally derived to assess psychopathic traits on the ratings by parents and teachers in preadolescent children. Frick later developed a self-report scale. The self-report version of the APSD has been successfully used to differentiate subgroups of juvenile offenders in other adolescent samples [140, 141].

5.3. The Child Psychopathy Scale (CPS)

The Child Psychopathy Scale (CPS) [142] is based on the PCL-R similar to the APSD. However, the items were drawn from the Child Behavior Checklist (CBCL) and the California Child Q-Set (CSQ). CPS contains 13 brief scales and the number of items representing each scale ranges from 2 to 7. [142].

5.4. The Youth Psychopathic Traits Inventory (YPI) and Child Version (YPI-CV)

The Youth Psychopathic Traits Inventory (YPI) [62] is a self-report psychopathy instrument theoretically based on the PCL-R. The YPI includes 10 scales constructed to measure 10 core personality traits associated with psychopathy. Each scale is composed of five items. Youths apply to them on a 4-point Likert scale. This measure is used for ages 12 and older [62].

The Youth Psychopathic Traits Inventory—Child version was developed by van Baardewijket al. to measure psychopathic traits in 9- to 12-year olds. They found that psychopathic traits can be measured reliably and meaningfully through self-report and that the YPI-CV is potentially a useful instrument [143].

5.5. The Hare P-SCAN: Research Version

Similar to the other measures discussed in this section, the Hare P-SCAN: Research Version is a screening device that draws its conceptual basis and its factor structure from the PCL-R. This 90-item questionnaire is scored on the "0–2" and items are grouped into "interpersonal," "affective," and "lifestyle" factors. Although age ranges are not specifically stated, the authors' references indicate that the P-SCAN is used for individuals aged 13 and older [144].

5.6. Child Problematic Traits Inventory (CPTI)

It is a new teacher-rated instrument to assess psychopathic personality from age 3 to 12 years. The CPTI items designed on three factors: "a Grandiose-Deceitful Factor, a Callous-Unemotional factor, and an Impulsive-Need for Stimulation factor." All of the factors showed reliability in

Instrument	Developed by	Structure and age
Psychopathy Checklist—Youth Version	Forth, Kosson, & Hare, 2003	A clinician-rated scale is used for adolescents aged 13–18 years
Antisocial Process Screening Device	Frick & Hare [140]	This measure was designed to measure psychopathy in children aged 6–12 years. It is completed by teachers or parents, rather than by self-report or interview with the young people themselves
The Child Psychopathy Scale	Lynam [142]	A parent/teacher-rated scale designed to assess psychopathy in late childhood and early adolescence
The Youth Psychopathic Traits Inventory	Andershed et al. [62]	A self-report, 50-item scale designed for young people of 12 years or older
The Youth Psychopathic Traits Inventory – Child version	Van Baardewijk et al. [143]	It was developed by van Baardewijk et al. to measure psychopathic traits in 9- to 12-year olds
The Hare P-SCAN: Research Version	Hare and Hervé [149]	P-SCAN is used for individuals aged 13 and older
Child Problematic Traits Inventory	Colins et al. [145]	It is a new teacher-rated instrument to assess psychopathic personality from age 3 to 12

Table 2. Current instruments for assessing psychopathy in children and adolescents.

internal consistency and external validity. The all of CPTI factors was a stronger predictor for showing that psychopathic personality construct in early childhood. In conclusion, the CPTI seems to be reliably and validly assessment tool for psychopathic traits in adolescence and adulthood [145].

The instruments for assessing of psychopathy in childhood and adolescence were listed in **Table 2**.

6. Comorbid disorders

The disorders frequently co-occurring with CD include various forms of depression, anxiety, substance use/abuse, and attention problems [146]. But psychopathic traits could be differentiated from CD about comorbid disorders.

In researches about comorbidity, Myers et al. have investigated the relations between psychopathy and Axis I and II psychopathology and delinquent behaviors in 30 psychiatrically hospitalized male and female adolescents. These authors found significant relations between psychopathy and CD, delinquent behaviors, substance abuse, and narcissistic personality disorder. Moreover, Myers et al. emphasized that psychopathic youth had multiple personality problems and they met diagnoses for many of the personality disorders [147].

More recently, Epstein et al. investigated the discriminant validity of psychopathy and mental disorders in a sample of 60 male adolescent adjudicated delinquents who were remanded for treatment. They found relations between adolescent psychopathy and alcohol dependence and substance dependence but not anxiety or depression [148]. Salekin et al. found that CD, ODD, ADHD, adjustment disorder, and substance abuse all correlated highly with the psychopathy scales. They showed also significant correlations across all three psychopathy scales were found for substance abuse, panic disorder, social phobia, and separation anxiety [37].

Bauer and Kosson examined 80 detained adolescent girls and reported that psychopathy was significantly associated with having a greater number of psychiatric diagnoses, and these coexisting disorders include alcohol dependence (61%), drug dependence (72%), ADHD (71%), dysthymia (22%), depression (52%), and PTSD (19%), even after removing CD from their analyses [149].

We need more detailed information about comorbidity and further research is needed regarding the relation between Axis I disorders and the facets of psychopathy with larger samples.

7. Prognosis

It is now well established that the most chronic and severe patterns of antisocial behavior are initiated early in life.

Therefore, understanding the development and stability of psychopathic personality from early childhood to adulthood may well be one of the most important missions for research aimed to understand the determinants of severe and long-lasting criminal behavior. Gretton et al. collected the file data of adolescent offenders and found that higher levels of psychopathic traits predicted an increased likelihood of violent offending 10 years later [150]. CU traits measured at school age predict antisocial and criminal behavior in adulthood, even after controlling for severity and onset of CD [151]. However, a notable longitudinal study found that psychopathic traits measured at age 13 were moderately stable to age 24, despite different informants and assessment instruments used across the two age periods [152].

Consistently with previous research, in the Pittsburgh Youth Study, psychopathy was assessed with the CPS and they were assessed with CPS at 12–13 years of age, which included both a high-risk group with disruptive behavior problems and a normative comparison group and they found that behavior problems were the most frequent, severe, aggressive, and temporally stable delinquent offenders in boys with high scores on the CPS [153].

In a notable study, Frick et al. examined psychopathy over a 4-year period and this sample included groups of children who, at baseline, were "(a) high on both CU traits and a measure of conduct problems; (b) high on CU traits, low on conduct problems; (c) high on conduct problems, low on CU traits; and (d) low on both measures." They found that "youth who originally had a lower score on psychopathic traits were less likely to have increasing scores over time." Youth with higher levels of conduct problems and lower levels of positive parenting (youth report) were more likely to have stable psychopathy scores. [154].

Waller et al. showed that adoptive mother observed positive parenting buffered the risk posed by early child fearlessness to later callous-unemotional behaviors [155].

These findings are interesting in that "they suggest that levels of psychopathic traits have the potential to change over time and may even be influenced by identifiable predictors."

Consistent with a growing literature showing that positive parenting—including warmth, responsivity, and praise—predict callous-unemotional behaviors, and this type of gene-environment interaction suggests that parent-child temperament pathways could also be moderated by caregiving quality [116, 156].

8. Treatment

The few studies that have examined the performance of youth with psychopathic features in treatment settings have found these youth to be more apt to disrupt the treatment and make less progress than youth with fewer psychopathic features [157–159]. Of the studies about treatment that compared the outcome of treatment for youths with conduct problems with and without elevated levels of CU traits, most of the studies reported that the group high on CU traits showed poorer treatment outcomes and treatment noncompliance. Specifically, several studies of adolescents with higher psychopathic or CU traits were demonstrated that adolescents were less compliance in treatment and poorer institutional adjustment and were more likely to reoffend after treatment [157, 160–162]. Similarly, in inpatient psychiatric settings, children (ages 7–11) with elevated levels of CU traits had longer length of stay and experienced more physically restrictive interventions during hospitalization [163]. In a school-aged sample of children enrolled in a summer treatment program for externalizing behavior problems, children with children conduct problems and CU traits responded less well to behavior therapy alone than children with conduct problems without CU traits [164] and less improvement in social skills and problem-solving skills when compared to children with CP alone [162]. Hawes and Dadds also found that boys with CU displayed lower treatment response to behavioral parent training and were particularly less responsive to time-outs [165].

When treatment strategies were investigated, McDonald et al. found that a parenting intervention successfully reduced levels of psychopathy-related traits among children aged 4–9 and that these effects were mediated by a reduction in levels of harsh and inconsistent parenting by mothers [166].

Kolko et al. conducted a randomized controlled trial of an intervention for 6- to 11-year-old children with conduct problems, in which one group was served through community settings (e.g., home, school, and neighborhood) and the other through a clinic. The intervention in both groups included parent training and other treatment methods such as family therapy and cognitive-behavioral therapy for the children. The results indicated that features of psychopathy were reduced in both groups of children, and the reductions were maintained over a 3-year follow-up period. Importantly, this study provides evidence that child psychopathic features can improve over time [167].

Specifically, once a reward-oriented response set has been established, children with elevated CU traits are slower to respond to punishment than children with normative levels of CU traits or children with high levels of anxiety. Thus, parenting practices that seek to encourage positive behavior through reinforcement or through other positive aspects of the parent-child relationship (e.g., fostering parental warmth, parent-child cooperation, positive reinforcement for appropriate child behaviors) may be particularly important for this group of children because of the focus on positive reinforcement rather than punishment [168].

In the recent study, the associations of both positive (i.e., warm and responsive) and negative (i.e., harsh and inconsistent) aspects of parenting with callous-unemotional (CU) traits and conduct problems in kindergarten students were tested, and they found that all three positive parenting variables (parental warmth, positive reinforcement, and parent-child cooperation and communication) were significantly negatively associated with CU trait levels. However, only parental warmth remained significantly negatively correlated with the level of CU traits after controlling the level of conduct problems. Thus, parental warmth may be particularly relevant for the development of CU traits [169]. This aspect of the parent-child relationship has been considered critical for the development of empathy, guilt, and other prosocial emotions, especially in children who have temperamental characteristics (e.g., low fear) that may interfere with the normal development of these emotions [170, 171]. Interventions that have focused on increasing parental warmth and increasing parents' use of positive reinforcement have led to reductions in the level of CU traits in young children [172, 173].

As a new treatment option, recent research has showed that omega-3 essential fatty acids supplementation could be an effective treatment for improving youth psychopathic behavior in the long term. Omega-3 has been known to be important for healthy brain development in children [174, 175] and low levels have been implicated in poor cognitive performance and behavior in children [176]. Another recent randomized controlled study was reported that omega-3 supplementation improved in callous-unemotional traits in 8- to 16-year-old children 6 months after the treatment ended. Additionally, "the parents of children receiving omega-3 supplementation showed a significant long-term reduction in their own psychopathic behavior." They suggested that reduction in parental psychopathy accounted for the improvement in their children's CU traits [177].

In conclusion, we concluded that there are some important points about treatment. First, given that children with CU traits start to show conduct problems early in their development and there are numerous interventions that have proven effective in treating early emerging conduct problems, early intervening of childhood-onset conduct problems were should be an important aim for preventing later serious aggression and antisocial behavior [178]. Second, in older children with severe antisocial behaviors, the most successful interventions are comprehensive and individualized interventions [179]. Researches on this area could help to guide these individualized interventions. For example, interventions that aim on anger control may be more effective for children within the childhood-onset pathway who do not have CU traits but who often show emotional problems. Treatment interventions such as to teach parents the ways to foster empathic concern in their child or help the child develop cognitive perspective-taking skills that aim to improve early in the parent-child relationship and they may be more effective for children with CU traits. Especially, later in development, reward-oriented response style attempt to motivate children through appealing to their self-interest may be more effective for this group rather than punishment-oriented strategies [180].

Author details

Merve Cikili Uytun

Address all correspondence to: mervecikili@yahoo.com

Department of Child and Adolescent Psychiatry, Sivas City Hospital, Sivas, Turkey

References

[1] Cooke DJ, Michie C. Refining the construct of psychopathy: Towards a hierarchical model. Psychological Assessment. 2001;**13**(2):171-188

[2] Harris GT, Rice ME, Cormier CA. Length of detention in matched groups of insanity acquittees and convicted offenders. International Journal of Law and Psychiatry. 1991;**14**(3):223-236

[3] Hare RD. The Hare Psychopathy Checklist-Revised. 2nd ed. NorthTonawanda, NY: Multi-Health Systems; 2003

[4] Dolan M. Psychopathic personality in young people. Advances in Psychiatric Treatment. 2004;**10**(6):466-473

[5] Douglas KS, Vincent GM, Edens JF. Risk for criminal recidivism: The role of psychopathy. In: Patrick CJ, editor. Handbook of Psychopathy. New York, USA: Guilford Press; 2006. pp. 533-555

[6] Leistico AM, Salekin RT, DeCoster J, Rogers R. A large-scale meta-analysis relating the hare measures of psychopathy to antisocial conduct. Law and Human Behavior. 2008;**32**(1):28-45

[7] Patrick CJ. Getting to the heart of psychopathy. In: Hervé H, Yuille JC, editors. The Psychopath: Theory, Research, and Practice. Mahwah (NJ): Lawrence Erlbaum Associates, Inc; 2007. pp. 207-252

[8] Hart SD HR. Psychopathy: Assessment and association with criminal conduct. In: Stoff DM, Breiling J, Maser J, editors. Handbook of Antisocial Behavior. New York: Wiley; 1997. pp. 22-35

[9] Moffitt TE, Caspi A, Dickson N, Silva P, Stanton W. Childhood-onset versus adolescent-onset antisocial conduct problems in males: Natural history from ages 3 to 18 years. Development and Psychopathology. 1996;**8**(02):399-424

[10] Lynam DR. Early identification of the fledgling psychopath: Locating the psychopathic child in the current nomenclature. Journal of Abnormal Psychology. 1998;**107**(4):566

[11] Hart SD, Kropp PR, Hare RD. Performance of male psychopaths following conditional release from prison. Journal of Consulting and Clinical Psychology. 1988;**56**(2):227

[12] Association AP. Diagnostic and Statistical Manual (DSM-III). Washington, DC: American Psychiatric Association; 1980

[13] Quay H. Patterns of delinquent behavior. In: Quay H, editor. Handbook of Juvenile Delinquency. New York: Wiley; 1987. pp. 118-138

[14] Rogeness GA, Javors MA, Pliszka SR. Neurochemistry and child and adolescent psychiatry. Journal of the American Academy of Child and Adolescent Psychiatry. 1992;**31**(5):765-781

[15] Frick PJ. Extending the construct of psychopathy to youth: Implications for understanding, diagnosing, and treating antisocial children and adolescents. Canadian Journal of Psychiatry. Revue Canadienne de Psychiatrie. 2009;**54**(12):803-812

[16] Association AP. Diagnostic and Statistical Manual (DSM-III-R). Washington, DC: American Psychiatric Association; 1987

[17] Frick PJ, Ellis M. Callous-unemotional traits and subtypes of conduct disorder. Clinical Child and Family Psychology Review. 1999;**2**(3):149-168

[18] Frick PJ, O'Brien BS, Wootton JM, McBurnett K. Psychopathy and conduct problems in children. Journal of Abnormal Psychology. 1994;**103**(4):700-707

[19] Lahey BB, Loeber R, Quay HC, Frick PJ, Grimm J. Oppositional defiant and conduct disorders: Issues to be resolved for DSM-IV. Journal of the American Academy of Child and Adolescent Psychiatry. 1992;**31**(3):539-546

[20] Lilienfeld SO, Waldman ID. The relation between childhood attention-deficit hyperactivity disorder and adult antisocial behavior reexamined: The problem of heterogeneity. Clinical Psychology Review. 1990;**10**(6):699-725

[21] Waschbusch DA. A meta-analytic examination of comorbid hyperactive-impulsive-attention problems and conduct problems. Psychological Bulletin. 2002;**128**(1):118-150

[22] Poulin F, Boivin M. Reactive and proactive aggression: Evidence of a two-factor model. Psychological Assessment. 2000;**12**(2):115

[23] Salmivalli C, Nieminen E. Proactive and reactive aggression among school bullies, victims, and bully-victims. Aggressive Behavior. 2002;**28**(1):30-44

[24] Dodge KA, Pettit GS. A biopsychosocial model of the development of chronic conduct problems in adolescence. Developmental Psychology. 2003;**39**(2):349

[25] Lemerise EA, Arsenio WF. An integrated model of emotion processes and cognition in social information processing. Child Development. 2000;**71**(1):107-118

[26] Cornell DG, Warren J, Hawk G, Stafford E, Oram G, Pine D. Psychopathy in instrumental and reactive violent offenders. Journal of Consulting and Clinical Psychology. 1996;**64**(4):783-790

[27] Woodworth M, Porter S. In cold blood: Characteristics of criminal homicides as a function of psychopathy. Journal of Abnormal Psychology. 2002;**111**(3):436-445

[28] Salekin RT. Psychopathy in children and adolescents: Key issues in conceptualization and assessment. In: Patrick JC, editor. Handbook of Psychopathy. New York, NY: Guilford Press; 2006. pp. 389-414

[29] Hare RD, Neumann CS. Psychopathy as a clinical and empirical construct. Annual Review of Clinical Psychology 2008;**4**:217-246

[30] Frick PJ, Dickens C. Current perspectives on conduct disorder. Current Psychiatry Reports. 2006;**8**(1):59-72

[31] Frick PJ, Marsee MA, Patrick C. Psychopathy and developmental pathways to antisocial behavior in youth. In: Patrick JC, editor. Handbook of Psychopathy. New York: Guilford Press; 2006. p. 353-374

[32] Frick PJ, White SF. Research review: The importance of callous-unemotional traits for developmental models of aggressive and antisocial behavior. Journal of Child Psychology and Psychiatry, and Allied Disciplines 2008;**49**(4):359-375

[33] Frick PJ, Stickle TR, Dandreaux DM, Farrell JM, Kimonis ER. Callous-unemotional traits in predicting the severity and stability of conduct problems and delinquency. Journal of Abnormal Child Psychology. 2005;**33**(4):471-487

[34] Association AP. Diagnostic and Statistical Manual (DSM-5). Washington, DC: American Psychiatric Association; 2013

[35] Costello EJ, Angold A. Developmental psychopathology and public health: Past, present, and future. Development and Psychopathology. 2000;**12**(4):599-618

[36] Webster-Stratton C, Hammond M. Conduct problems and level of social competence in Head Start children: Prevalence, pervasiveness, and associated risk factors. Clinical Child and Family Psychology Review. 1998;**1**(2):101-124

[37] Salekin RT, Leistico AM, Neumann CS, DiCicco TM, Duros RL. Psychopathy and comorbidity in a young offender sample: Taking a closer look at psychopathy's potential importance over disruptive behavior disorders. Journal of Abnormal Psychology. 2004;**113**(3):416-427

[38] Hare RD, Hart SD, Harpur TJ. Psychopathy and the DSM-IV criteria for antisocial personality disorder. Journal of Abnormal Psychology. 1991;**100**(3):391-398

[39] Forth AE, Burke HC. Psychopathy in adolescence: Assesment, Violence and Developmental Precursors. In: Cooke DJ, Forth AE, Hare RD editors. Psychopathy: Theory, Research and Implications for Society. Portugal: Springer; 1998. pp.205-229

[40] Brandt GT, Norwood AE, Ursano RJ, Wain H, Jaccard JT, Fullerton CS, et al. Psychiatric morbidity in medical and surgical patients evacuated from the Persian Gulf War. Psychiatric Services. 1997;**48**(1):102-104

[41] Viding E, McCrory E, Seara-Cardoso A. Psychopathy. Current Biology. 2014;**24**(18): R871-R874

[42] Bezdjian S, Raine A, Baker LA, Lynam DR. Psychopathic personality in children: Genetic and environmental contributions. Psychological Medicine. 2011;**41**(3):589-600

[43] Blonigen DM, Hicks BM, Krueger RF, Patrick CJ, Iacono WG. Continuity and change in psychopathic traits as measured via normal-range personality: A longitudinal-biometric study. Journal of Abnormal Psychology. 2006;**115**(1):85-95

[44] Larsson H, Andershed H, Lichtenstein P. A genetic factor explains most of the variation in the psychopathic personality. Journal of Abnormal Psychology. 2006;**115**(2):221-230

[45] Taylor J, Loney BR, Bobadilla L, Iacono WG, McGue M. Genetic and environmental influences on psychopathy trait dimensions in a community sample of male twins. Journal of Abnormal Child Psychology. 2003;**31**(6):633-645

[46] Bezdjian S, Tuvblad C, Raine A, Baker LA. The genetic and environmental covariation among psychopathic personality traits, and reactive and proactive aggression in childhood. Child Development. 2011;**82**(4):1267-1281

[47] Viding E, Frick PJ, Plomin R. Aetiology of the relationship between callous-unemotional traits and conduct problems in childhood. The British Journal of Psychiatry. Supplement 2007;**49**:s33-s38

[48] Waldman ID, Tackett JL, Van Hulle CA, Applegate B, Pardini D, Frick PJ, et al. Child and adolescent conduct disorder substantially shares genetic influences with three socioemotional dispositions. Journal of Abnormal Psychology. 2011;**120**(1):57-70

[49] Viding E, Blair RJ, Moffitt TE, Plomin R. Evidence for substantial genetic risk for psychopathy in 7-year-olds. Journal of Child Psychology and Psychiatry, and Allied Disciplines 2005;**46**(6):592-597

[50] Viding E, Jones AP, Frick PJ, Moffitt TE, Plomin R. Heritability of antisocial behaviour at 9: Do callous-unemotional traits matter? Developmental Science. 2008;**11**(1):17-22

[51] Rijsdijk FV, Viding E, De Brito S, Forgiarini M, Mechelli A, Jones AP, et al. Heritable variations in gray matter concentration as a potential endophenotype for psychopathic traits. Archives of General Psychiatry. 2010;**67**(4):406-413

[52] Viding E, Hanscombe KB, Curtis CJ, Davis OS, Meaburn EL, Plomin R. In search of genes associated with risk for psychopathic tendencies in children: A two-stage genome-wide association study of pooled DNA. Journal of Child Psychology and Psychiatry, and Allied Disciplines 2010;**51**(7):780-788

[53] Hirata Y, Zai CC, Nowrouzi B, Beitchman JH, Kennedy JL. Study of the catechol-o-methyltransferase (COMT) gene with high aggression in children. Aggressive Behavior. 2013;**39**(1):45-51

[54] Gogos JA, Morgan M, Luine V, Santha M, Ogawa S, Pfaff D, et al. Catechol-O-methyltransferase-deficient mice exhibit sexually dimorphic changes in catecholamine levels and behavior. Proceedings of the National Academy of Sciences. 1998;**95**(17):9991-9996

[55] Fowler T, Langley K, Rice F, van den Bree MB, Ross K, Wilkinson LS, et al. Psychopathy trait scores in adolescents with childhood ADHD: The contribution of genotypes affecting MAOA, 5HTT and COMT activity. Psychiatric Genetics. 2009;**19**(6):312-319

[56] Beitchman JH, Zai CC, Muir K, Berall L, Nowrouzi B, Choi E, et al. Childhood aggression, callous-unemotional traits and oxytocin genes. European Child & Adolescent Psychiatry. 2012;**21**(3):125-132

[57] Hirata Y, Zai CC, Nowrouzi B, Shaikh SA, Kennedy JL, Beitchman JH. Possible association between the prolactin receptor gene and callous-unemotional traits among aggressive children. Psychiatric Genetics. 2016;**26**(1):48-51

[58] Binder EB. The role of FKBP5, a co-chaperone of the glucocorticoid receptor in the pathogenesis and therapy of affective and anxiety disorders. Psychoneuroendocrinology 2009;**34**:S186-S195

[59] Bevilacqua L, Carli V, Sarchiapone M, George DK, Goldman D, Roy A, et al. Interaction between FKBP5 and childhood trauma and risk of aggressive behavior. Archives of General Psychiatry. 2012;**69**(1):62-70

[60] Holz NE, Buchmann AF, Boecker R, Blomeyer D, Baumeister S, Wolf I, et al. Role of FKBP5 in emotion processing: Results on amygdala activity, connectivity and volume. Brain Structure and Function. 2015;**220**(3):1355-1368

[61] White MG, Bogdan R, Fisher PM, Munoz K, Williamson DE, Hariri AR. FKBP5 and emotional neglect interact to predict individual differences in amygdala reactivity. Genes, Brain and Behavior 2012;**11**(7):869-878

[62] Andershed H, Gustafson SB, Kerr M, Stattin H. The usefulness of self-reported psychopathy-like traits in the study of antisocial behaviour among non-referred adolescents. European Journal of Personality. 2002;**16**(5):383-402

[63] Frick PJ, Lilienfeld SO, Ellis M, Loney B, Silverthorn P. The association between anxiety and psychopathy dimensions in children. Journal of Abnormal Child Psychology. 1999;**27**(5):383-392

[64] Blair RJ. Neurobiological basis of psychopathy. The British Journal of Psychiatry: the Journal of Mental Science 2003;**182**:5-7

[65] Barker ED, Oliver BR, Viding E, Salekin RT, Maughan B. The impact of prenatal maternal risk, fearless temperament and early parenting on adolescent callous-unemotional traits: A 14-year longitudinal investigation. Journal of Child Psychology and Psychiatry, and Allied Disciplines 2011;**52**(8):878-888

[66] Waller R, Gardner F, Viding E, Shaw DS, Dishion TJ, Wilson MN, et al. Bidirectional associations between parental warmth, callous unemotional behavior, and behavior problems in high-risk preschoolers. Journal of Abnormal Child Psychology. 2014;**42**(8):1275-1285

[67] Dadds MR, Allen JL, McGregor K, Woolgar M, Viding E, Scott S. Callous-unemotional traits in children and mechanisms of impaired eye contact during expressions of love: A treatment target? Journal of Child Psychology and Psychiatry, and Allied Disciplines 2014;**55**(7):771-780

[68] Waller R, Hyde LW, Grabell AS, Alves ML, Olson SL. Differential associations of early callous-unemotional, oppositional, and ADHD behaviors: Multiple domains within early-starting conduct problems? Journal of Child Psychology and Psychiatry, and Allied Disciplines 2015;**56**(6):657-666

[69] Barry CT, Frick PJ, Killian AL. The relation of narcissism and self-esteem to conduct problems in children: A preliminary investigation. Journal of Clinical Child and Adolescent Psychology. 2003;**32**(1):139-152

[70] Kerig PK, Stellwagen KK. Roles of callous-unemotional traits, narcissism, and Machiavellianism in childhood aggression. Journal of Psychopathology and Behavioral Assessment. 2010;**32**(3):343-352

[71] Lau KS, Marsee MA. Exploring narcissism, psychopathy, and Machiavellianism in youth: Examination of associations with antisocial behavior and aggression. Journal of Child and Family Studies. 2013;**22**(3):355-367

[72] Marsh AA, Finger EC, Mitchell DG, Reid ME, Sims C, Kosson DS, et al. Reduced amygdala response to fearful expressions in children and adolescents with callous-unemotional traits and disruptive behavior disorders. The American Journal of Psychiatry. 2008;**165**(6):712-720

[73] Jones AP, Laurens KR, Herba CM, Barker GJ, Viding E. Amygdala hypoactivity to fearful faces in boys with conduct problems and callous-unemotional traits. The American Journal of Psychiatry. 2009;**166**(1):95-102

[74] White SF, Marsh AA, Fowler KA, Schechter JC, Adalio C, Pope K, et al. Reduced amygdala response in youths with disruptive behavior disorders and psychopathic traits: Decreased emotional response versus increased top-down attention to nonemotional features. The American Journal of Psychiatry. 2012;**169**(7):750-758

[75] Lozier LM, Cardinale EM, VanMeter JW, Marsh AA. Mediation of the relationship between callous-unemotional traits and proactive aggression by amygdala response to fear among children with conduct problems. JAMA Psychiatry. 2014;**71**(6):627-636

[76] Viding E, Fontaine NM, McCrory EJ. Antisocial behaviour in children with and without callous-unemotional traits. Journal of the Royal Society of Medicine. 2012;**105**(5):195-200

[77] Sebastian CL, McCrory EJ, Cecil CA, Lockwood PL, De Brito SA, Fontaine NM, et al. Neural responses to affective and cognitive theory of mind in children with conduct problems and varying levels of callous-unemotional traits. Archives of General Psychiatry. 2012;**69**(8):814-822

[78] Finger EC, Marsh A, Blair KS, Majestic C, Evangelou I, Gupta K, et al. Impaired functional but preserved structural connectivity in limbic white matter tracts in youth with conduct disorder or oppositional defiant disorder plus psychopathic traits. Psychiatry Research. 2012;**202**(3):239-244

[79] Finger EC, Marsh AA, Mitchell DG, Reid ME, Sims C, Budhani S, et al. Abnormal ventromedial prefrontal cortex function in children with psychopathic traits during reversal learning. Archives of General Psychiatry. 2008;**65**(5):586-594

[80] Wallace GL, White SF, Robustelli B, Sinclair S, Hwang S, Martin A, et al. Cortical and subcortical abnormalities in youths with conduct disorder and elevated callous-unemotional traits. Journal of the American Academy of Child and Adolescent Psychiatry. 2014;**53**(4):456-465 e1

[81] De Brito SA, Mechelli A, Wilke M, Laurens KR, Jones AP, Barker GJ, et al. Size matters: Increased grey matter in boys with conduct problems and callous-unemotional traits. Brain: A Journal of Neurology. 2009;**132**(Pt 4):843-852

[82] Fairchild G, Hagan CC, Walsh ND, Passamonti L, Calder AJ, Goodyer IM. Brain structure abnormalities in adolescent girls with conduct disorder. Journal of Child Psychology and Psychiatry, and Allied Disciplines 2013;**54**(1):86-95

[83] Pardini DA, Raine A, Erickson K, Loeber R. Lower amygdala volume in men is associated with childhood aggression, early psychopathic traits, and future violence. Biological Psychiatry. 2014;**75**(1):73-80

[84] Ermer E, Kahn RE, Salovey P, Kiehl KA. Emotional intelligence in incarcerated men with psychopathic traits. Journal of Personality and Social Psychology. 2012;**103**(1):194-204

[85] Cope LM, Ermer E, Nyalakanti PK, Calhoun VD, Kiehl KA. Paralimbic gray matter reductions in incarcerated adolescent females with psychopathic traits. Journal of Abnormal Child Psychology. 2014;**42**(4):659-668

[86] Finger EC, Marsh AA, Blair KS, Reid ME, Sims C, Ng P, et al. Disrupted reinforcement signaling in the orbitofrontal cortex and caudate in youths with conduct disorder or oppositional defiant disorder and a high level of psychopathic traits. The American Journal of Psychiatry. 2011;**168**(2):152-162

[87] White SF, Brislin S, Sinclair S, Fowler KA, Pope K, Blair RJ. The relationship between large cavum septum pellucidum and antisocial behavior, callous-unemotional traits and psychopathy in adolescents. Journal of Child Psychology and Psychiatry, and Allied Disciplines 2013;**54**(5):575-581

[88] Zhou J, Yao N, Fairchild G, Zhang Y, Wang X. Altered hemodynamic activity in conduct disorder: A resting-state FMRI investigation. PLoS One. 2015;**10**(3):e0122750

[89] Zhou J, Yao N, Fairchild G, Cao X, Zhang Y, Xiang YT, et al. Disrupted default mode network connectivity in male adolescents with conduct disorder. Brain Imaging and Behavior. 2016;**10**(4):995-1003

[90] Sonuga-Barke EJ, Castellanos FX. Spontaneous attentional fluctuations in impaired states and pathological conditions: A neurobiological hypothesis. Neuroscience & Biobehavioral Reviews. 2007;**31**(7):977-986

[91] Uytun MC, Karakaya E, Oztop DB, Gengec S, Gumus K, Ozmen S, et al. Default mode network activity and neuropsychological profile in male children and adolescents with attention deficit hyperactivity disorder and conduct disorder. Brain Imaging and Behavior. 2016: 1-10

[92] Swanson J, Baler RD, Volkow ND. Understanding the effects of stimulant medications on cognition in individuals with attention-deficit hyperactivity disorder: A decade of progress. Neuropsychopharmacology: Official Publication of the American College of Neuropsychopharmacology. 2011;**36**(1):207-226.

[93] Frick PJ, Ray JV, Thornton LC, Kahn RE. Can callous-unemotional traits enhance the understanding, diagnosis, and treatment of serious conduct problems in children and adolescents? A comprehensive review. Psychological Bulletin. 2014;**140**(1):1-57

[94] Fisher L, Blair RJ. Cognitive impairment and its relationship to psychopathic tendencies in children with emotional and behavioral difficulties. Journal of Abnormal Child Psychology. 1998;**26**(6):511-519

[95] Frick PJ, Cornell AH, Bodin SD, Dane HE, Barry CT, Loney BR. Callous-unemotional traits and developmental pathways to severe conduct problems. Developmental Psychology. 2003;**39**(2):246-260

[96] Centifanti LC, Modecki K. Throwing caution to the wind: Callous-unemotional traits and risk taking in adolescents. Journal of Clinical Child and Adolescent Psychology: The Official Journal for the Society of Clinical Child and Adolescent Psychology, American Psychological Association, Division 53. 2013;**42**(1):106-119

[97] Blair RJ, Colledge E, Mitchell DG. Somatic markers and response reversal: Is there orbitofrontal cortex dysfunction in boys with psychopathic tendencies? Journal of Abnormal Child Psychology. 2001;**29**(6):499-511

[98] Dadds MR, Gale N, Godbee M, Moul C, Pasalich DS, Fink E, et al. Expression and regulation of attachment-related emotions in children with conduct problems and callous-unemotional traits. Child Psychiatry and Human Development. 2016;**47**(4):647-656

[99] Pardini D. Perceptions of social conflicts among incarcerated adolescents with callous-unemotional traits: 'you're going to pay. It's going to hurt, but I don't care'. Journal of Child Psychology and Psychiatry, and Allied Disciplines. 2011;**52**(3):248-255

[100] Pardini DA, Lochman JE, Frick PJ. Callous/unemotional traits and social-cognitive processes in adjudicated youths. Journal of the American Academy of Child and Adolescent Psychiatry. 2003;**42**(3):364-371

[101] Stickle TR, Kirkpatrick NM, Brush LN. Callous-unemotional traits and social information processing: Multiple risk-factor models for understanding aggressive behavior in antisocial youth. Law and Human Behavior. 2009;**33**(6):515-529

[102] Chabrol H, van Leeuwen N, Rodgers RF, Gibbs JC. Relations between self-serving cognitive distortions, psychopathic traits, and antisocial behavior in a non-clinical sample of adolescents. Personality and Individual Differences. 2011;**51**(8):887-892

[103] Dadds MR, Cauchi AJ, Wimalaweera S, Hawes DJ, Brennan J. Outcomes, moderators, and mediators of empathic-emotion recognition training for complex conduct problems in childhood. Psychiatry Research. 2012;**199**(3):201-207

[104] Jones AP, Happe FG, Gilbert F, Burnett S, Viding E. Feeling, caring, knowing: Different types of empathy deficit in boys with psychopathic tendencies and autism spectrum disorder. Journal of Child Psychology and Psychiatry, and Allied Disciplines 2010;**51**(11):1188-1197

[105] Pardini DA, Byrd AL. Perceptions of aggressive conflicts and others' distress in children with callous-unemotional traits: 'I'll show you who's boss, even if you suffer and I get in trouble'. Journal of Child Psychology and Psychiatry, and Allied Disciplines 2012;**53**(3):283-291

[106] Dadds MR, Hawes DJ, Frost AD, Vassallo S, Bunn P, Hunter K, et al. Learning to 'talk the talk: The relationship of psychopathic traits to deficits in empathy across childhood. Journal of Child Psychology and Psychiatry, and Allied Disciplines 2009;**50**(5): 599-606

[107] Stellwagen KK, Kerig PK. Ringleader bullying: Association with psychopathic narcissism and theory of mind among child psychiatric inpatients. Child Psychiatry and Human Development. 2013;**44**(5):612-620

[108] Christian RE, Frick PJ, Hill NL, Tyler L, Frazer DR. Psychopathy and conduct problems in children: II. Implications for subtyping children with conduct problems. Journal of the American Academy of Child and Adolescent Psychiatry. 1997;**36**(2):233-241

[109] Loney B, Frick P, Ellis M, Coy M. Intelligence, psychopathy, and antisocial behaviour. Journal of Psychopathology and Behavioural Assessment. 1998;**20**:231-247

[110] Salekin RT, Neumann CS, Leistico AM, Zalot AA. Psychopathy in youth and intelligence: An investigation of Cleckley's hypothesis. Journal of Clinical Child and Adolescent Psychology: The Official Journal for the Society of Clinical Child and Adolescent Psychology, American Psychological Association, Division 53. 2004;**33**(4):731-742

[111] Waschbusch DA, Walsh TM, Andrade BF, King S, Carrey NJ. Social problem solving, conduct problems, and callous-unemotional traits in children. Child Psychiatry and Human Development. 2007;**37**(4):293-305

[112] Delisi M, Vaughn M, Beaver KM, Wexler J, Barth AE, Fletcher JM. Fledgling Psychopathy in the Classroom: ADHD Subtypes Psychopathy, and Reading Comprehension in a Community Sample of Adolescents. Youth Violence and Juvenile Justice. 2011;**9**(1):43-58

[113] Vaughn MG, DeLisi M, Beaver KM, Wexler J, Barth A, Fletcher J. Juvenile psychopathic personality traits are associated with poor reading achievement. The Psychiatric Quarterly. 2011;**82**(3):177-190

[114] Edens JF, Skopp NA, Cahill MA. Psychopathic features moderate the relationship between harsh and inconsistent parental discipline and adolescent antisocial behavior. Journal of Clinical Child and Adolescent Psychology: The Official Journal for the Society of Clinical Child and Adolescent Psychology, American Psychological Association, Division 53. 2008;**37**(2):472-476

[115] Hipwell AE, Pardini DA, Loeber R, Sembower M, Keenan K, Stouthamer-Loeber M. Callous-unemotional behaviors in young girls: Shared and unique effects relative to conduct problems. Journal of Clinical Child and Adolescent Psychology: The Official Journal for the Society of Clinical Child and Adolescent Psychology, American Psychological Association, Division 53. 2007;**36**(3):293-304

[116] Pasalich DS, Dadds MR, Hawes DJ, Brennan J. Do callous-unemotional traits moderate the relative importance of parental coercion versus warmth in child conduct problems? An observational study. Journal of Child Psychology and Psychiatry, and Allied Disciplines 2011;**52**(12):1308-1315

[117] Waller R, Gardner F, Hyde LW, Shaw DS, Dishion TJ, Wilson MN. Do harsh and positive parenting predict parent reports of deceitful-callous behavior in early childhood? Journal of Child Psychology and Psychiatry. 2012;**53**(9):946-953

[118] Pardini DA, Loeber R. Interpersonal callousness trajectories across adolescence: Early social influences and adult outcomes. Criminal Justice and Behavior. 2008;**35**(2):173-196

[119] Kochanska G, Kim S, Boldt LJ, Yoon JE. Children's callous-unemotional traits moderate links between their positive relationships with parents at preschool age and externalizing behavior problems at early school age. Journal of Child Psychology and Psychiatry, and Allied Disciplines 2013;**54**(11):1251-1260

[120] Waller R, Gardner F, Shaw DS, Dishion TJ, Wilson MN, Hyde LW. Callous-unemotional behavior and early-childhood onset of behavior problems: The role of parental harshness and warmth. Journal of Clinical Child and Adolescent Psychology: The Official Journal for the Society of Clinical Child and Adolescent Psychology, American Psychological Association, Division 53. 2015;**44**(4):655-667

[121] Kroneman LM, Hipwell AE, Loeber R, Koot HM, Pardini DA. Contextual risk factors as predictors of disruptive behavior disorder trajectories in girls: The moderating effect of callous-unemotional features. Journal of Child Psychology and Psychiatry, and Allied Disciplines 2011;**52**(2):167-175

[122] Bakermans-Kranenburg MJ, van IJzendoorn MH. The first 10,000 Adult Attachment Interviews: Distributions of adult attachment representations in clinical and non-clinical groups. Attachment & Human Development. 2009;**11**(3):223-263

[123] Dadds MR, Jambrak J, Pasalich D, Hawes DJ, Brennan J. Impaired attention to the eyes of attachment figures and the developmental origins of psychopathy. Journal of Child Psychology and Psychiatry, and Allied Disciplines 2011;**52**(3):238-245

[124] Campbell MA, Porter S, Santor D. Psychopathic traits in adolescent offenders: An evaluation of criminal history, clinical, and psychosocial correlates. Behavioral Sciences & the Law. 2004;**22**(1):23-47

[125] Bernstein DP, Stein JA, Handelsman L. Predicting personality pathology among adult patients with substance use disorders: Effects of childhood maltreatment. Addictive Behaviors. 1998;**23**(6):855-868

[126] Jaffee SR, Caspi A, Moffitt TE, Taylor A. Physical maltreatment victim to antisocial child: Evidence of an environmentally mediated process. Journal of Abnormal Psychology. 2004;**113**(1):44-55

[127] Krischer MK, Sevecke K. Early traumatization and psychopathy in female and male juvenile offenders. International Journal of Law and Psychiatry. 2008;**31**(3):253-262

[128] Muñoz LC, Kerr M, Besic N. The peer relationships of youths with psychopathic personality traits a matter of perspective. Criminal Justice and Behavior. 2008;**35**(2):212-227

[129] Barker ED, Salekin RT. Irritable oppositional defiance and callous unemotional traits: Is the association partially explained by peer victimization? Journal of Child Psychology and Psychiatry, and Allied Disciplines 2012;**53**(11):1167-1175

[130] Goldweber A, Dmitrieva J, Cauffman E, Piquero AR, Steinberg L. The development of criminal style in adolescence and young adulthood: Separating the lemmings from the loners. Journal of Youth and Adolescence. 2011;**40**(3):332-346

[131] Kimonis ER, Frick PJ, Barry CT. Callous-unemotional traits and delinquent peer affiliation. Journal of Consulting and Clinical Psychology. 2004;**72**(6):956-966

[132] Anastassiou-Hadjicharalambous X, Warden D. Physiologically-indexed and self-perceived affective empathy in conduct-disordered children high and low on callous-unemotional traits. Child Psychiatry and Human Development. 2008;**39**(4):503-517

[133] de Wied M, van Boxtel A, Matthys W, Meeus W. Verbal, facial and autonomic responses to empathy-eliciting film clips by disruptive male adolescents with high versus low callous-unemotional traits. Journal of Abnormal Child Psychology. 2012;**40**(2):211-223

[134] Fung MT, Raine A, Loeber R, Lynam DR, Steinhauer SR, Venables PH, et al. Reduced electrodermal activity in psychopathy-prone adolescents. Journal of Abnormal Psychology. 2005;**114**(2):187-196

[135] Isen J, Raine A, Baker L, Dawson M, Bezdjian S, Lozano DI. Sex-specific association between psychopathic traits and electrodermal reactivity in children. Journal of Abnormal Psychology. 2010;**119**(1):216-225

[136] Kimonis ER, Frick PJ, Skeem JL, Marsee MA, Cruise K, Munoz LC, et al. Assessing callous-unemotional traits in adolescent offenders: Validation of the inventory of callous-unemotional traits. International Journal of Law and Psychiatry. 2008;**31**(3):241-252

[137] Stadler C, Kroeger A, Weyers P, Grasmann D, Horschinek M, Freitag C, et al. Cortisol reactivity in boys with attention-deficit/hyperactivity disorder and disruptive behavior problems: The impact of callous unemotional traits. Psychiatry Research. 2011;**187**(1-2): 204-209

[138] Kotler JS, McMahon RJ. Assessment of child and adolescent psychopathy. In: Salekin RT, Lynam DR, editor. Handbook of Child and Adolescent Psychopathy. New York: The Guilford Press.; 2010. pp. 79-109

[139] Forth AE. Hare Psychopathy Checklist, Youth Version (PCL: YV). In: Thomas Grisso, Gina Vincent, Daniel Seagrave, editors. Mental Health Screening and Assessment in Juvenile Justice. New York: Guildford press; 2005. pp. 324-339

[140] Frick PJ, Hare RD. Antisocial Process Screening Device: APSD. Toronto: Multi-Health Systems; 2001

[141] Loney BR, Frick PJ, Clements CB, Ellis ML, Kerlin K. Callous-unemotional traits, impulsivity, and emotional processing in adolescents with antisocial behavior problems. Journal of Clinical Child and Adolescent Psychology: The Official Journal for the Society of Clinical Child and Adolescent Psychology, American Psychological Association, Division 53. 2003;**32**(1):66-80

[142] Lynam DR. Pursuing the psychopath: Capturing the fledgling psychopath in a nomological net. Journal of Abnormal Psychology 1997;**106**:425-438

[143] van Baardewijk Y, Stegge H, Andershed H, Thomaes S, Scholte E, Vermeiren R. Measuring psychopathic traits in children through self-report. The development of the Youth Psychopathic Traits Inventory-Child Version. International Journal of Law and Psychiatry. 2008;**31**(3):199-209

[144] Hare R, Hervé H. Hare P-Scan: Research Version. Toronto, ON: Multi-Health Systems Inc.; 1999

[145] Colins OF, Andershed H, Frogner L, Lopez-Romero L, Veen V, Andershed AK. A new measure to assess psychopathic personality in children: The Child Problematic Traits Inventory. Journal of Psychopathology and Behavioral Assessment. 2014;**36**(1):4-21

[146] Hinshaw SP, Zupan BA. Assessment of antisocial behavior in children and adolescents. In: Barkley EJMRA, editor. Child Psychopathology. New York: Guilford Press; 1997. pp. 36-50

[147] Myers WC, Burket RC, Harris HE. Adolescent psychopathy in relation to delinquent behaviors, conduct disorder, and personality disorders. Journal of Forensic Sciences. 1995;**40**(3):435-439

[148] Epstein M, Douglas D, Poythress N, Spain S, Falkenbach D, editors. A discriminant study of juvenile psychopathy and mental disorders. Conference of the American Psychology-Law Society, Austin, TX; March 2002

[149] Bauer D, Kosson D, editors. Psychopathy in incarcerated females: Prevalence rates and individual differences in personality and behavior. Conference of the American Psychology-Law Society, New Orleans, LA; March 2000

[150] Gretton HM, Hare RD, Catchpole RE. Psychopathy and offending from adolescence to adulthood: A 10-year follow-up. Journal of Consulting and Clinical Psychology. 2004;**72**(4):636-645

[151] McMahon RJ, Witkiewitz K, Kotler JS, Conduct problems prevention research G. Predictive validity of callous-unemotional traits measured in early adolescence with respect to multiple antisocial outcomes. Journal of Abnormal Psychology. 2010;**119**(4):752-763

[152] Lynam DR, Caspi A, Moffitt TE, Loeber R, Stouthamer-Loeber M. Longitudinal evidence that psychopathy scores in early adolescence predict adult psychopathy. Journal of Abnormal Psychology. 2007;**116**(1):155-165

[153] Loeber R, Farrington DP, Stouthamer-Loeber M, Moffitt TE, Caspi A, Lynam D. Male mental health problems, psychopathy, and personality traits: Key findings from the first 14 years of the Pittsburgh Youth Study. Clinical Child and Family Psychology Review. 2001;**4**(4):273-297

[154] Frick PJ, Kimonis ER, Dandreaux DM, Farell JM. The 4-year stability of psychopathic traits in non-referred youth. Behavioral Sciences & the Law. 2003;**21**(6):713-736

[155] Waller R, Trentacosta CJ, Shaw DS, Neiderhiser JM, Ganiban JM, Reiss D, et al. Heritable temperament pathways to early callous-unemotional behaviour. The British Journal of Psychiatry: the Journal of Mental Science. 2016;**209**(6):475-482

[156] Waller R, Gardner F, Hyde LW. What are the associations between parenting, callous-unemotional traits, and antisocial behavior in youth? A systematic review of evidence. Clinical Psychology Review. 2013;**33**(4):593-608

[157] Falkenbach DM, Poythress NG, Heide KM. Psychopathic features in a juvenile diversion population: Reliability and predictive validity of two self-report measures. Behavioral Sciences & the Law. 2003;**21**(6):787-805

[158] O'Neill ML, Lidz V, Heilbrun K. Adolescents with psychopathic characteristics in a substance abusing cohort: Treatment process and outcomes. Law and Human Behavior. 2003;**27**(3):299-313

[159] Spain SE, Douglas KS, Poythress NG, Epstein M. The relationship between psychopathic features, violence and treatment outcome: The comparison of three youth measures of psychopathic features. Behavioral Sciences & the Law. 2004;**22**(1):85-102

[160] Rogers R, Johansen J, Chang JJ, Salekin RT. Predictors of adolescent psychopathy: Oppositional and conduct-disordered symptoms. The Journal of the American Academy of Psychiatry and the Law. 1997;**25**(3):261-271

[161] Gretton HM, McBride M, Hare RD, O'Shaughnessy R, Kumka G. Psychopathy and recidivism in adolescent sex offenders. Criminal Justice and Behavior. 2001;**28**(4):427-449

[162] Haas SM, Waschbusch DA, Pelham WE, Jr., King S, Andrade BF, Carrey NJ. Treatment response in CP/ADHD children with callous/unemotional traits. Journal of Abnormal Child Psychology. 2011;**39**(4):541-552

[163] Stellwagen KK, Kerig PK. Relation of callous-unemotional traits to length of stay among youth hospitalized at a state psychiatric inpatient facility. Child Psychiatry and Human Development. 2010;**41**(3):251-261

[164] Waschbusch DA, Carrey NJ, Willoughby MT, King S, Andrade BF. Effects of methylphenidate and behavior modification on the social and academic behavior of children with disruptive behavior disorders: The moderating role of callous/unemotional traits. Journal of Clinical Child and Adolescent Psychology: The Official Journal for the Society of Clinical Child and Adolescent Psychology, American Psychological Association, Division 53. 2007;**36**(4):629-644

[165] Hawes DJ, Dadds MR. The treatment of conduct problems in children with callous-unemotional traits. Journal of Consulting and Clinical Psychology. 2005;**73**(4):737-741

[166] McDonald R, Dodson MC, Rosenfield D, Jouriles EN. Effects of a parenting intervention on features of psychopathy in children. Journal of Abnormal Child Psychology. 2011;**39**(7):1013-1023

[167] Kolko DJ, Dorn LD, Bukstein OG, Pardini D, Holden EA, Hart J. Community vs. clinic-based modular treatment of children with early-onset ODD or CD: A clinical trial with 3-year follow-up. Journal of Abnormal Child Psychology. 2009;**37**(5):591-609

[168] O'Brien BS, Frick PJ. Reward dominance: Associations with anxiety, conduct problems, and psychopathy in children. Journal of Abnormal Child Psychology. 1996;**24**(2):223-240

[169] Clark JE, Frick PJ. Positive parenting and callous-unemotional traits: their association with school behavior problems in young children. Journal of Clinical Child and Adolescent Psychology. 2016;**53**:1-13

[170] Cornell AH, Frick PJ. The moderating effects of parenting styles in the association between behavioral inhibition and parent-reported guilt and empathy in preschool children. Journal of Clinical Child and Adolescent Psychology. 2007;**36**(3):305-318

[171] Dadds MR, Moul C, Cauchi A, Hawes DJ, Brennan J. Replication of a ROBO2 polymorphism associated with conduct problems but not psychopathic tendencies in children. Psychiatric Genetics. 2013;**23**(6):251-254

[172] Hawes DJ, Dadds MR, Frost AD, Hasking PA. Do childhood callous-unemotional traits drive change in parenting practices? Journal of Clinical Child and Adolescent Psychology: The Official Journal for the Society of Clinical Child and Adolescent Psychology, American Psychological Association, Division 53. 2011;**40**(4):507-518

[173] Kimonis ER, Bagner DM, Linares D, Blake CA, Rodriguez G. Parent Training outcomes among young children with callous-unemotional conduct problems with or at-risk for developmental delay. Journal of Child and Family Studies. 2014;**23**(2):437-448

[174] Ryan AS, Astwood JD, Gautier S, Kuratko CN, Nelson EB, Salem N, Jr. Effects of long-chain polyunsaturated fatty acid supplementation on neurodevelopment in childhood: A review of human studies. Prostaglandins, Leukotrienes, and Essential Fatty Acids 2010;**82**(4-6):305-314

[175] Schuchardt JP, Huss M, Stauss-Grabo M, Hahn A. Significance of long-chain polyunsaturated fatty acids (PUFAs) for the development and behaviour of children. European Journal of Pediatrics. 2010;**169**(2):149-164

[176] Montgomery P, Burton JR, Sewell RP, Spreckelsen TF, Richardson AJ. Low blood long chain omega-3 fatty acids in UK children are associated with poor cognitive performance and behavior: A cross-sectional analysis from the DOLAB study. PLoS One. 2013;**8**(6):e66697

[177] Raine A, Portnoy J, Liu J, Mahoomed T, Hibbeln JR. Reduction in behavior problems with omega-3 supplementation in children aged 8-16 years: A randomized, double-blind, placebo-controlled, stratified, parallel-group trial. Journal of Child Psychology and Psychiatry, and Allied Disciplines 2015;**56**(5):509-520

[178] Eyberg SM, Nelson MM, Boggs SR. Evidence-based psychosocial treatments for children and adolescents with disruptive behavior. Journal of Clinical Child & Adolescent Psychology. 2008;**37**(1):215-237

[179] Henggeler SW, Schoenwald SK, Borduin CM, Rowland MD, Cunningham PB. Multisystemic Therapy for Antisocial Behavior in Children and Adolescents. New York: Guildford Press; 2009

[180] Frick PJ. Developmental pathways to conduct disorder. Child and Adolescent Psychiatric Clinics of North America. 2006;**15**(2):311-331, vii

Chapter 3

The Problem of Adolescent Psychopathy: The Downward Extension of Adult Psychopathy

Margarida Simões and Rui Abrunhosa Gonçalves

Additional information is available at the end of the chapter

http://dx.doi.org/10.5772/intechopen.68963

Abstract

With this theoretical review, we intend to understand the relationship between adolescent psychopathy and adult psychopathy, taking into account three fundamental questions: (1) the conceptualization of personality, in other words, knowing the extent to which it makes sense to speak about a structured and defined personality in adolescents; (2) the notion of disorder quite present in the stage of adolescent development; (3) and finally, whether the previously alleged disorders are stable identities or if they have temporal continuity, extending into adult life. We are aware that there is no unanimity or consensus regarding the essential core of psychopathy, that is, it presents itself in distinct ways that make it difficult to configure it in taxonomical or dimensional terms of the personality, ignoring much about its etiology, these uncertainties, end up to be translated into a major openness to the study of pre-adult population. Thus, the study of adolescent and juvenile psychopathy will depend a lot on how much we know about adult psychopathy. This does not imply that we do not carry out studies of a longitudinal and measuring nature through psychometric instruments that allow us to clarify the way this syndrome manifests itself and develops throughout life, taking into account the Big Five.

Keywords: psychopathy, adolescence, adulthood, personality, development

1. Introduction

In a study about psychopathy in adolescence, it is inevitable to address the question whether there are, in this age group, individuals with this disorder or, at least to speak more prudently, whether we can safely identify, adolescent individuals with psychopathic traits. This problem was unnoticed for many years because the investigations, up to recent date, were initially oriented toward those who manifested expressed behaviors of psychopathy, that is, repeat offenders and highly violent adults, revealing high levels of callous-unemotional traits. Among these investigations, only sporadically, there are descriptions of young psychopaths, as in Bowlby's study [1] on juvenile offenders, but who would not at the time have followers.

In fact, the issue of juvenile and adolescent psychopathy only began to be seriously discussed just over 20 years ago, especially since the investigations of Frick et al. [2] and Lynam [3], coincident with the time when courts began to pronounce sentences on defendants from these age groups on the basis of psychopathy diagnoses (mostly in Canada but also in the US; see Ref. Frick [4]). This controversy emerged especially in the early twenty-first century, with the publishing of various numbers of prestigious journals entirely dedicated to this subject (e.g., *Law and Human Behavior*, 26 (2), 2002 and *Behavioral Sciences and the Law*, 21, 2003), considering divergent views, with some authors being skeptical against the existence of this personality disorder (PD) before adult life as opposed to those defending the opposite view. The most skeptical [5] argued that many of the typical psychopathic traits were specific of their own or inherent to development in adolescence, and therefore, it was questionable that true psychopaths could be identified in this population stratum, or, in an even more radical way, it was assured that there are no juvenile psychopaths and adolescents, because, in a general way, personality has not fully stabilized until this age, and therefore, we cannot speak about personality disorders before adult life [6].

Basically, this emphasized controversy has been based on three major and compelling questions for those who propose to investigate psychopathy before adulthood, without having the ambition to bring things to a closure, namely: *The first question* relates to the *conceptualization of personality* itself. It is questioned in the debate the legitimacy to speak about the *personality of an adolescent*, as it would correspond to something that would only have its *stable structure with the emergence of adulthood*. The *second question* relates to the notion of disorder, or stating Wallon [7], it means knowing whether *the adolescent disorders are "turbulences" inherent to their development, or if they are they likely to have a clinical-forensic status*. Finally, *the third question* relates to whether the alleged *disorders are stable entities and if they have temporal continuity, extending into adult life*. In the following chapters, we will answer these three questions.

1.1. The personality in childhood and adolescence—continuity and development

In popular psychology (folk psychology), in Bruner's interpretation [8], personality exists before the age of 18. The parents of the children routinely refer to their children's personality, whether they use that word, or use another word that is equivalents in the current language, for example, "temperament" or "way of being."

The accumulated evidence in the last 10 years about the structure and development of juvenile and adolescent personality has shown that it has very similar characteristics to adult personality. The temperament traits organize themselves in a similar way to adult personality traits, as it has been repeatedly highlighted by Caspi and his co-workers [9, 10]. Therefore, we can speak of a temperament *organization*, whose analysis was started by Thomas and Chess, in 1963, within a longitudinal study on temperament traits stability in babies and children, the New York Longitudinal Study [11]. The original model of these authors distinguished

http://dx.doi.org/10.5772/intechopen.68963

nine temperament traits, which would be present since early childhood. More recent models, resulting from questionnaires and observation protocols, achieved, by factorial analysis, less temperamental traits, generally 6 or 7. Thus, Caspi et al. [9] list the following six traits, as being typical of contemporary research: level of activity; positive emotions/pleasure (distress); irritable/anger/frustration (distress); fearful/escape from new situations (including social situations); tranquility (tendency to remain calm) and ability to concentrate/persist. It is possible to match, at least partially, these six temperamental traits with the higher-order personality traits as a result from adult research, the *Big Five*: Extraversion, Neuroticism, Agreeableness, Conscientiousness and Openness to Experience [12]. For example, several factorial analyzes of questionnaires, adjective lists, and California Child Q-Set produced factors similar to the Big Five and some of their subfactors (so-called second-order factors), in children and adolescents (see Ref. [10, p. 307]). As a result of these studies, Caspi and Shiner [10] elaborated a proposal for a taxonomy of first- and second-order personality traits of children and adolescents, which will represent the personality of these age groups and is, as can be seen in **Table 1**, structurally identical to that of adults. This does not mean that there are no differences among children, adolescents, and adults as regards the delicate organization (i.e., in terms of the second-order traits) of the personality. It is certain that some temperamental characteristics of children do not find accurate match in the next age stages (e.g., it is the case of irritability), and it is seen equally that the factorial composition of the *Big Five* is, in some cases, defined by different items in the instruments used in children and adults [13]. However, in general, we can draw from these results the conclusion that it is not only legitimate to speak of personality before adulthood [10, p. 307], since the age of 3. We may or may not designate this personality by the word temperament, but it is also appropriate to say that in structural terms, the constituent elements of the adult personality have been available since childhood. But it cannot be inferred from it that the organization of personality is unchangeable. As Caspi et al. said, "although children exhibit traits that are remarkably similar to those found in adults,

First-order traits	Extraversion (E)	Neuroticism (N)	Conscientiousness (C)	Agreeableness (A)	Openness to experience (O)
First-order traits	Sociability	Fear	Attention	Prosocial	Intellect
	Energy/Level of activity	Anxiety	Self-control	Tendencies	Creativity
		Sadness	Achievement striving	Antagonism	Curiosity
			Orderliness	Obstinacy	
	Low E + N	N + Low A	C + A		
	Social inhibition	Anger/Irritability	Responsibility		
		Alienation/ suspicious			

Adapted from Caspi and Shiner [10]. *Note: the second-order traits referred to in the lower part of the table saturate in both indicated first-order traits*

Table 1. A taxonomy of personality traits in children and adolescents.

researchers should be aware of developmental differences in the manifestation of these traits; for example, the traits may be less coherent in early infancy" [9, p. 456].

The empirical analysis of stability versus life-long personality change can be made in the perspective of Caspi et al. using three types of studies, called *differential* measurement, *mean-level* measurement and *ipsative* measurement [10]. Although different, these three types of study provide results that are complementary and whose integration is essential in order to have a complete and rigorous representation of the degree of personality stability.

Differential studies, of a longitudinal nature, compare, for each temperament or personality trait, and on several successive moments, the related positions of a group of individuals, using statistical procedures of test-retest (rank-order correlation). The objective is to know, for each measured trait (e.g., anxiety in children and young adolescents, or its equivalent in older adolescents and young adults), if these individuals maintain, in those successive moments, the same positions. As an example, if, in a group of 100 individuals, the result of a three-year-old child in a measure of sociability reveals her as the most sociable, and then at 12 years of age, its result will maintain her in the same position, we will say that there is differential stability, regardless of whether this result may vary in absolute value.

The so-called middle-level studies, meanwhile, aim to measure the average absolute value (*mean-level*) of one or several first- and second-order traits in a given population, in order to determine the extent to which the different aspects of personality retain, throughout life, and especially in moments considered as transition, the same average operative expressiveness. In other words, we want to determine to what extent the overall structure of personality, expressed in terms of the absolute values of its different components, varies over time for the population as a whole. While it is desirable that these studies be longitudinal, thus ensuring that temporal fluctuations in trait intensity are measured in the same individuals, there are other investigations that use a cross-sectional methodology, measuring at the same time the mean level of traits in different cohorts.

Both the differential and the mean-level investigations have as a common element the fact of comparing a group of individuals regarding the results (relative and absolute) obtained in one or several components of the personality. That is, there are studies that seek to determine continuity (stability), in this case, the statistical distribution of the results of a group or, inferentially, the population of individuals in these traits (the variables), ignoring their specific configuration for each individual. They are, therefore, investigations *focused on the variables.* On the other hand, ipsative longitudinal studies in Block's (1971) *are people-centered* as they seek to determine how, in each person, the personality structure—defined by the results of each trait or component—varies over time. For this purpose, this internal structure is measured in two or more moments of time by Q-Sort type methodology, obtaining an overall coherence index (by Q-Sort correlation) that represents the degree to which the individuals of a sample will vary over time.

After analyzing the methodologies, we will present the main empirical conclusions pertaining to these three types of studies. To that end, we will rely mainly on some recent meta-analyzes performed by Roberts and DelVecchio (2000), and by Roberts, Walton, and Viechtbauer (2006), as well as two excellent syntheses produced by Caspi and his collaborators (Caspi et al., 2005; Caspi & Shiner, 2006).

1.2. Differential Continuity (*rank-order*) of personality

The meta-analysis that Roberts and Delvecchio (2000) [14] carried out, taking as reference organization the Big Five, considered 152 differential personality studies, allowing the following conclusion: (a) from childhood to adulthood, test-retest correlations (rank-order) are moderate, with an average value after correction for the reduction of 0.40; (b) stability tends to increase with age, from 0.41 in childhood to 0, 55 at age 30, reaching a maximum value of 0.74 between ages 50 and 70 (reviewed values); (c) the stability decreases as measurement is more spaced in time; (d) it does not vary between traits; (e) neither with the assessment method; and (f) nor by gender. These results show, according to Caspi et al. [9, p. 466–467], that the magnitude of personality stability is overall impressive and only exceeded, in all psychology, by the stability of cognitive ability measures and interests referring specially to adolescence, as well as the fact, "that the level of stability increases in an approximately linear way through adolescence and first stage of young adulthood."

1.3. Stability and change in mean-level

In an investigation led by Roberts et al. [15], 92 studies were reviewed on stability and change of mean-level of personality domains, organized according to *Big Five* and its features, throughout life. The results of that meta-analysis showed that: (a) pertaining to *extraversion*, the side of social dominance (assertiveness, dominance) increased since adolescence until middle age, especially in the first stage of adulthood (20–40 years of age), whereas the side of social vitality (sociability, talkativeness) increased in adolescence and decreased in adulthood; (b) in *agreeableness* and *conscientiousness*, the results increased in the first stage of adulthood and middle age; (c) the neuroticism traits decreased equally during adult life (20 years upwards); and (d) *openness* to *experience* traits increased in adolescence and in the first stage of adulthood, and decreased in old age.

A surprising result shows that the most mean-level personality traits change occurs during the first stage of adult life between 20 and 40, Caspi and Shiner [10, p. 337], suggested that the investigation of the personality maturation mechanisms should be focused at this age.

1.4. Ipsative stability and change

There are very few longitudinal studies that have used Block's (1971) Q-Sort Method to measure the internal change in personality structure of individuals. This is disappointing, because of the above-mentioned differential and mid-continuity research, concentrating on the overall variance of traits in groups or populations, tend to encapsulate the cases of individual variation that occur in them. That is to say, no one tells us what percentage of individuals in these groups exhibits internal structural stability, and how many are those with moderate or marked variations. It is not clear, how many people in each cohort are stable and how many are not. In Block's (1971) study, this methodology was used in a pioneering way, with great differences in the degree of personality stability among individuals. Although the Q-Sort correlation showed high stability for the groups as a whole—0.70 between childhood and the end of adolescence and 0.50 between this and adult life—these results concealed the enormous variability between individuals. For example, the intraindividual Q-Sort correlation, that is, for each individual, varied between median negative values and positive values so high that they were only limited by the measurement error margin. This means that in each cohort, there are people whose trait structure, measured by the Q-Sort correlation over time, is invariant, and others in which the personality seems to undergo severe structural inversions. Similar results were obtained in more recent studies, with intraindividual variations between 0.44 and 0.90 (Asendorpf & van Aken, 1991; Ozer & Gjerde, 1989). An interesting conclusion of these studies is that intraindividual stability is not a result of chance but seems to be associated with positive personality traits such as sociability, emotional control, and conscientiousness, which tend to increase the resilience of individuals to the difficulties of life (Caspi & Shiner, 2006).

In Block's study [16], the Q-sort techniques were used in a pioneering way, and it was established that there were major differences in personality stability rank among individuals. Although the Q-Sort correlation showed high stability for groups as a whole—0.70 between childhood and late adolescence and 0.50 between this and adult life, these results hid the huge variability between individuals. One interesting conclusion of these studies is that the intraindividual stability is not a random result, but it seems to be associated with positive personality traits, such as sociability, emotional control, and conscientiousness, which tend to increase the resiliency of the individuals facing difficulties in life [10].

1.5. Personality disorders (PDs) existence and stability before adult life

As we mentioned before, a first question that arises for those who approach the problem of psychopathy in adolescence is to know whether there are personality disorders (PDs) before adult life. In a very influential article, Seagrave and Grisso [5] draw particular attention to the attention that the physician must have in order not to confuse traits inherent to the development, and therefore transitional, of adolescence itself with the constellation of proto-psychopath deviant personality traits. That is, to identify true positives, not false positives, as they say. This is a reasonable requirement, and, in our view, it is not being contested. However, as we saw earlier, some authors went even further, stating that there are reasons to believe that in adolescence, there is not even a consolidated personality, and consequently, that there can be no personality disorder. This is the case of Hart, et al. [6, p. 242] when they affirm that there is "no consensus among developmental psychopathologists that personality disorder as a generic class of psychopathology does not even exist in childhood and adolescence" (242). To this extent, it seems to us clear that this matter, whether it is possible to speak of personality disorders before adult life, in what precise terms, from what age, and with what empirical evidence, clinical examination is warranted.

The DSM-V defines a personality disorder as being

> *"a persistent pattern of inner experience and behavior that deviates markedly from the expectations of the individual's culture, is diffuse and inflexible, begins in adolescence or early adulthood, it is stable over time and leads to suffering or injury."* [17, p. 645]

Now, apparently, the DSM recognizes the possibility of personality disorders before adulthood, more specifically in adolescence. Admittedly, there is no clear reference to what stage of adolescence or what possible disorders may occur. But in practice, as Kernberg et al. (2000, p. 6) state that "for personal and theoretical reasons, physicians have been reluctant to diagnose a personality disorder in children and adolescents" [18, p. 6]. These authors state the reasons, more practical than substantial, for this reluctance.

> *"fear of putting young people prematurely on a negative label that will affect their self-image and jeopardize them in the future, the refusal by insurance companies to bear health expenses in these cases, on the grounds that such diseases are not officially cataloged, and finally, the conviction, expressed by many professionals, that the personality is not yet sufficiently consolidated to justify such a diagnosis."* [18, p. 6]

Aspects of personal functioning implied in the future constitution of a distinct personality are also early distinguishable, at least from the end of basic schooling, or even earlier, with unique styles of thought and linguistic intelligence, as well as persistence and operability, widely attested by empirical studies, of a style of bonding that, established in childhood, may appear as a striking element for certain so-called personality pathologies. The question does not, therefore, seem to be whether there are personality disorders before adulthood and even before adolescence. In short, we believe that we have provided evidence that legitimizes us to adopt the point of view of the existence of personality disorders in adolescence, or that these are disorders defined by the lacking developmental framework.

However, these same authors consider the reasons described as unjustified. For them, "PDs in children, as in adults, can be reliably identified, correlated with other disorders of axes I and II, and show a pattern of persistence that makes their impact generalized and strict" [18, p. 14]. And they list a set of other reasons which, in their opinion, support their position: the very early existence (2 and 3 years of age) of self-consciousness of self, of a feeling of self and of the idea of the other as an empathic individual (resonant to the other).

As several authors argument (i.e., "e.g., see Ref. [19]."), what needs explanation is not the personality's mutability, but its opposite, that is, the fact that it presents a considerable degree of stability throughout life.

Sometimes we find in literature references to the extreme volatility of PDs in periods prior to adulthood, especially during adolescence. For example, see Ref. [20], in a longitudinal study with adolescents from a community population, reports not only a significant incidence of PDs but also a high percentage of cases with spontaneous remission after a short time (approximately 40%). Hart, Watt, and Vincent invoke these results to conclude that there is reason to "doubt the accuracy of the initial diagnosis" [6, p. 242]. Here, we are faced with a problem that escalates the study of PDs in these age groups: the method or procedure used to identify the pathology. Kernberg and his associates [18] point out that the complexity inherent to the personality construct, a dynamic cluster of traits and components, makes the diagnosis more dependent on the used procedures, at least partially explaining the sometimes enormous differences that we find in studies on the juvenile prevalence of these syndromes. To this extent, it will be much more difficult to diagnose a PD than an isolated trait of the constitutive temperament of that PD, or a pathology of Axis I. To do so, the physician must identify the pattern, often complex and fluid, and often idiosyncratic, of the multiplicity of traits and behaviors that constitute, by definition, the PD, and to interpret the meaning and operational value of these traits and behaviors in the context of the developmental situation in which they occur.

Although there is still much to discover about the formation and stability of the personality and its disorders along the lifespan of individuals, we are not being audacious if we conclude that a basis of evidence has gradually been established which will ensure that the personality itself, and its disorders which may be inherent to it are organized in the majority of individuals before adulthood, not to say that they are organized earlier; or enable to state that the constituent elements of the personality would already be available at a younger age. In this line of thought, for example, in an important longitudinal study that followed 1037 individuals from 3 to 21 years of age, Caspi (2000) showed an impressive continuity of temperamental traits throughout this period. In his opinion, it can start even before 3 years of age, stating that:

> *"The second year of life may be the crucial dividing line for predicting adult personality differences in adulthood because of the cognitive-emotional changes that take place during this period. During the second year of life, perceptual and cognitive changes allow the child to acquire the [notion of] permanence of objects and participate in symbolic games. Self-conscious emotions such as embarrassment and shame also begin to appear at this time These capacities may be necessary for children to form mental representations of their social world and to develop beliefs and expectations that are then confirmed by a reactive and more diverse social environment."* [21, p. 169]

1.6. The nature and stability of psychopathy in childhood and adolescence

The fact that most personality disorders can be built before adulthood does not mean that this is automatically true in the specific case of psychopathy. However, we can discuss with Lynam [22] that psychopathy is not, in itself, different from other PDs and therefore does not justify a particular a priori reservation regarding this pathology. Or, in the same sense, according to Seagrave and Grisso [5], the typical traits of psychopathy (impulsivity, a tendency toward deviant behavior, ethical relativism and egocentricity) are precisely those that tend to emerge during adolescence, although with an episodic intensity and transient nature.

In general, the authors agree that there is still a shortage of longitudinal studies on psychopathy.

The authors who affirm the existence of juvenile and adolescent psychopathy do not call into question the need to be especially cautious with the diagnosis of psychopathy applied to children and adolescents. They acknowledge that the label can have serious legal consequences [4] and that, given the present unresolved controversy over the treatability of this "pathology" [23, 24], these consequences could extend to the clinical domain. It is therefore ethically recommendable that any diagnosis of psychopathy, especially when applied to adolescents, will be supported by scientifically rigorous criteria [4]. Consequently, in general, these authors tend to avoid the designation of psychopaths when referring to pre-adults, preferring rather that of "individuals with psychopathic traits." For their part, the arguments invoked to speak of juvenile psychopathy are various. Lynam [3] coined the term "incipient psychopath" *"Fledgling psychopath"* to designate children with behavioral problems (CP) who simultaneously exhibited high levels of hyperactive-impulsive-attention problems (HIA) and who, in their opinion, were "affected by a virulent variant of behavioral disorder (CD) which will be more appropriately described as fledgling psychopathy" [3, p. 209] and has recently been described by DSMV [17] as presenting "characteristics necessary for the specifier" "with Limited Prosocial Emotions" with callous and unemotional traits; a search for strong emotions;

http://dx.doi.org/10.5772/intechopen.68963

audacity and insensitivity to punishments. Since then, several researchers have sought to accumulate empirical evidence to determine the characteristics of these young people and whether this category is stable and can be identified with adult psychopathy. It is, in our view, possible to address the multiple reasons invoked to speak of juvenile psychopathy in the following categories:

(a) there is a remarkable stability in temperament and personality traits since adolescence, even since childhood, and in particular, in the callous and unemotional traits and emotional deficit traits that are typical of adult psychopathy;

(b) it is possible to map, according to statistically solid criteria, personality traits of psychopathy (adult and juvenile) in different profiles according to the Big Five model;

(c) there is a laboratory and neuropsychological evidence that suggests that psychopathy is associated with early anatomical and/or physiological dysfunction, possibly with a genetic substrate;

(d) the measurement of juvenile psychopathy by the available instruments shows us that the construct targeted by these instruments has content and factorial validity and is structurally similar to the construct measured by the instruments used with adult psychopaths, especially PCL-R.

Despite the recent nature of the subject, there are already, as we said, some reflections on these arguments [25–28]). The principal impression after reading these reflections is that, to quote one of them, "the evaluation of psychopathy in children and adolescents is a very important research area, and it is still in its childhood, and our knowledge about nature, stability, and consequences of juvenile psychopathy (…) is very limited "[26, p. 471]. We, therefore, think that it is useful to continue and enhance the research on this issue.

Most of the physicians who are confronted institutionally with heterogeneous groups of juvenile delinquents are liable to recognize, at least in some of these offenders, John Bowlby's description of fourteen of the 44 boys and girls whom he examined in 1944. The interest of this study will be, above all, in the fact that Bowlby identified in children—under the age of 12—the temperament traits that constitute the main subject of contemporary research on juvenile psychopathy: absence of affective bonds, to react emotionally, precocious and recurrence delinquency, instrumental violence, impulsivity, and superficial charm and deceptive intelligence. And, what is an important aspect, of distinguishing these young people from other aggressive juvenile delinquents, which he calls *Hyperthymics* [1]. And this is this difference that has, in some way, been one of the key reasons for considering the existence of juvenile psychopathy, isolating it from commonly associated disorders and seeking to give it its own entity.

To conclude, the Klingzell's study [29] shows the stability and change of psychopathic traits since childhood. Other authors, through their studies accomplished with community samples, showed that the stability of psychopathic traits could be found since childhood until adulthood, as well as, between the adolescence and adulthood [30, 31].

1.7. Nomological network similar to adult psychopathy

They have been identified by the PCL: YV (The Hare Psychopathy Checklist: Youth Version), and other assessment instruments of adolescent and juvenile psychopathy, some young adults with psychopathic traits, showing a coherent range of characteristics that differentiate them from the remaining juvenile offenders; similar characteristics to those which distinguish adult psychopaths from adults characterized as ASPD non-psychopaths, for example, callous and unemotional traits [32, 33]; the number of violent acts and the criminal versatility [34, 35]; the recidivism and criminal conduct persistence over the years [36–39]; the preference for the instrumental violence [40]; and the lack of positive results after the exposure to therapy [41].

These studies have repeatedly shown that the relationship between the results of psychopathy and the used criteria variables is predicted by the theory, thus reinforcing the idea of the existence of a subgroup of CD with psychopathic characteristics present in the specifier "with Limited Prosocial Emotions" (DSMV). This relationship has been pointed out as strong, persisting even when the PCL: YV or APSD traits constituting the antisocial factor are eliminated from the predictive equations of regression [40], which shows that the callous and unemotional traits and emotional deficit traits are sufficient to justify, in the current state of our knowledge, the use of the fledgling psychopathy feature as a possible characterizing syndrome of a distinct subgroup of young adults and adolescents with behavioral disorders.

1.8. Psychopathy and personality

In recent years, Donald Lynam has been developing an interesting research program on the relationship between psychopathy and personality structure. The central objective of this program is "not to discuss whether psychopathy is related to personality… [But rather] to gather evidence that psychopathy is personality" [Emphasis of the original]. That is, the basic premise … is that psychopathy can be understood as a particular constellation of basic personality traits … [42, p. 133–134], especially the basic traits recognized by most personality theorists [43]. The reference to this research program is important since, although most researches have been focused on adult psychopathy, Lynam and his colleagues tested the structural model of psychopathy with the structure of personality in samples with adolescents and found that this model was essentially identical to that of adults [22, 27].

Lyman's and collaborators research program resulted from the convergence of three research strategies:

(a) the performance of a meta-analysis [42] on the correlation between psychopathy and personality traits based on studies that allowed this comparison. That is, studies in which in the samples were available psychopathy results obtained with the application of PCL-R or other specific instruments and results pertaining to basic personality traits resulting from the application of standardized personality measures, namely NEO-PI-R from Costa and Mc Crae [44], Tellegen's Multidimensional Personality Questionnaire [45], and Eysenck's PEN [46]. Although different, these three personality models can be subsumed into a single model, which Lynam calls *the four major consensuals* (Consensual Big Four), which is composed of the following personality super dimensions: neuroticism, extraversion, pleasure, and conscientiousness.

(b) the translation of the PCL-R checklist in terms of the language of the structural models of personality, that is, the assignment of each of the 20 items of this checklist to one (or more) dimensions and second-order traits of those models and determination of its meaning (e.g., item number 1 of PCL-R, "superficial charm," was classified as low self-consciousness, a feature of Neuroticism, so it was defined as N).

(c) the description by recognized psychopathy experts of the typical traits of a psychopath in terms of the language of the structural models of personality [47] or a non-theoretical instrument such as Common Language California Child Q-Sort Version (CLQ) [22].

These three methods have produced results that converge with each other, allowing a general translation of the personality configuration typical of the psychopath in the language of the structural models of personality [42]. The resulting description varies according to the dimensions: an individual with low Pleasure (A) and high personal antagonism; the psychopath is "egocentric, suspicious, aggressive and does not care about others" [42, p. 139]. The Conscientiousness/Control (C) feature is also associated, in a negative sense, with psychopathy, showing the psychopathic individual as "not able to control himself and to adhere to traditional values and patterns of conduct" [42, p. 139]. Less clear were the results regarding Neuroticism (N) and Extraversion (E), where the relation of psychopathy to these higher-order personality dimensions seems to be more subtle depending on the second-order factors to be considered. The psychopath may have high values of hostility and impulsivity (two factors of N), but low values of self-consciousness (another factor of N), and high values of demand for exciting sensations (an E-factor) and low positive emotions and cordiality (another factor of E).

The importance of Lyman's research program in this context in the present chapter is renewed by the fact that, in one of the studies, Common Language Q-Sort (CLQ) has been used to characterize the "incipient psychopath" [22]. The juvenile psychopath portrait resulting from that study is similar to the one obtained with other methods and for adult population: "The incipient psychopath is extremely low in Agreeableness, extremely low in Conscientiousness and somehow low in Neuroticism" [41, p. 143]. These results were expressed according to the 10 most characteristic verbal descriptions and the 10 less descriptive descriptions of an incipient psychopath, which by its importance are reproduced in **Table 2**.

1.9. Factor structure of juvenile psychopathy measurement instruments

If in some way the structure of juvenile psychopathy proves to be in accordance with the structure of adult psychopathy, it is to be expected that this conformity will also be revealed in the factor structure of the instruments used to measure this "pathology" throughout life. More specifically, measurement instruments for juvenile psychopathy should reveal, for example, when applied to samples with adolescents, a structure semantically similar to that, which is obtained consistently with the classical instruments of adult psychopathy, and especially

Topic CLQ		Average	DP	Range	FFM Scale
Characteristic topics					
11	He tries to blame others for what he does	9.0	0.00	9–9	$A^- C^-$
22	He tries to make others do what he wants to, manipulating them. He uses his personal charm to get what he wants	8.5	0.76	7–9	A^-
65	When he wants something, he wants it now. He has difficulty waiting for the things he wants and what he likes	8.5	0.53	8–9	$A^- C^-$
20	He tries to take advantage of others	8.4	0.71	7–9	$A^- C^-$
13	He tries to see how far he can go. He goes over the limit and tries to bend the rules as far as possible.	8.3	0.71	7–9	$A^- C^-$
21	He tries to be the center of attention	8.0	1.07	6–9	$A^- C^-$
85	He is aggressive	8.0	0.76	7–9	$A^- C^-$
10	His friendships do not last long, he often changes friends	7.6	1.69	4–9	$A^- C^-$
91	His emotions do not seem to fit the situation	7.6	0.92	6–9	$A^- C^-$
93	He is bossy and tries to dominate others	7.6	0.74	6–8	A^-
Non-characteristic topics					
76	You can trust him, he is reliable	1.3	0.46	1–2	C^+
15	He shows concern to what is correct and what is not	1.9	0.99	1–4	$A^+ C^+$
62	He is obedient and does what he is told to	1.9	0.83	1–3	$A^+ C^+$
99	He thinks about what he is going to do, he uses his head before he does something or says something	1.9	0.83	1–3	C^+
9	He establishes solid and intimate relationships with other people	2.0	0.76	1–3	A^+
67	He plans ahead, he thinks before he does something, he "looks before he jumps"	2.0	0.93	1–3	C^+
23	He is nervous and fearsome	2.3	0.89	1–3	N^+
77	He feels insecure, he has a poor opinion of himself	2.4	1.19	1–4	N^+
2	He is kind and worries about others	2.5	1.60	1–5	A^+
3	He is a warm person and responds kindly to others	2.5	1.07	2–5	A^+

Adapted from Lynam [22]. Note: each topic is rated between 1 (extremely uncharacteristic) and 9 (extremely characteristic). A, C, and N are the domains of pleasure, conscientiousness, and neuroticism. As we have pointed out, the above-mentioned table clearly shows the most common features with emphasis on the expression of dominating others (e.g., topic 11: He tries to blame others or topic 22: He tries to make others do what he wants to, manipulating them), expressions that can be observed already in children, or that are like proto-behaviors (e.g., opposition phase, well-known challenge of developmentalists), and in adolescents.

Table 2. Characteristic and non-characteristic topics of the incipient psychopath according to the Common Language Q-Sort.

with PCL-R. In this respect, if it exists, it will be an additional argument in favor of the existence of adolescent psychopathy, with characteristics that allow us to identify it as an unequivocal precursor of adult psychopathy.

http://dx.doi.org/10.5772/intechopen.68963

There is currently a considerable range of studies on the psychometric characteristics of juvenile psychopathy measurement instruments. We will examine these instruments in detail later, so here we shall limit ourselves to summarizing their main aspects considered as the most relevant to the present problem. However, the issue is somehow complicated by the fact that the less recent investigations—let us say before 2001—use as a comparative model the traditional bi-factorial structure of PCL-R (with two factors, called Factor 1 = Interpersonal/ Affective and Factor 2 = Social Deviance) and the more recent tend to be aligned with Cooke et al. [48] proposal of a three-factor structure (composed of interpersonal, affective and lifestyle factors) or the proposal of Hare et al. [49, 51], which contemplates a fourth dimension related to the antisocial behavior itself. This fact does not facilitate the comparison between the two types of studies and their integration in the meta-analysis. It should also be said that the problems of the interpretation of the psychometric properties of the instruments of measurement of juvenile psychopathy are not substantially different from those with their adult counterparts, for example, the problem of the possible hierarchical, or first-order factorial, nature of the construct, as well as the problem of the true status of the items that operationalize the antisocial dimension (see the controversy between Hare and Cooke and Michie in Recent Handbook of Psychopathy, edited by Patrick [50, 48].

Forth and collaborates [52] report, in the PCL manual: YV (adapted version of PCL-R for adolescents), results of validation studies, which show that this instrument presents the same PCL-R factor structure, in particular, the structure in non-hierarchical four factors, which is the most recent proposal for this instrument of reference. The confirmatory factorial analysis was based on large samples of 5964 incarcerated adults and in 1631 adolescents. Comparative diagrammatic representations can be analyzed in Hare and Neumann [49, p. 77–78] and show, with small differences, an impressive coincidence in the structural representation between the two groups.

The three-factor model of Cooke and Michie has also been successfully replicated in PCL: YV [34, 53–55], unlike the original two-factor model [56]. These results with PCL: YV are especially significant as it is a checklist for adolescents derived from a checklist formulated for adults (PCL-R).

The similarity between the factor structures of the two instruments is, therefore, an indicator that adolescent psychopathy is a consistent construct.

Factor validation results for other instruments of application in juvenile and adolescent samples have been, however, less conclusive. In the case of APSD [57], which is also an adaptation of PCL-R for children between 6 and 12 years of age, some studies report having obtained two factors, similar to those of PCL-R [2, 58]. In the Frick, Bodin and Barry study [58], a three-factor structure was also obtained, but its isomorphism with that of PCL-R is doubtful. The authors report a factor of callous-unemotional and interpersonal deficit and another component, called impulsivity and behavior problems (I/CP), which unfolded in two factors, one of which (composed of seven items) reflects interpersonal aspects and which they called narcissism, and the other (consisting of five items) will measure impulsivity. On the other hand, in a study that used a self-filling variant of APSD, and aimed at adolescents [59], a trifactorial structure is considered appropriate. Another instrument that has been used with adolescents is the CPS (Childhood Psychopathy Scale), by Lynam [36], aimed at individuals between the ages of 6 and 17. A revised version, mCPS, and composed of 55 items, was recently presented [60]. This version has an autoresponder variant for teenagers. The structure of this scale is currently still little known, given the paucity of factorial validation studies. Salekin [28], however, refers to it as a promising instrument for measuring psychopathy. In general, the measurement instruments of juvenile and adolescent psychopathy provide the investigator a mixed background, except for PCL: YV, which seems to measure the same construct as PCL-R and with the same psychometric structure. The other instruments available differ significantly from PCL and its variants. Although we can say that there is systematically, a factor linked to callous-unemotional and another to impulsiveness, the status of antisocial behavior items is less clear. One possible explanation for this is that the life history of young people and adolescents is not enough to stabilize this factor, which depends on an accumulation of deviant experiences.

Another possibility is that there is a complex of behavioral traits that, being equally typical and normative of adolescence, confuse the specific antisociality of proto-psychopaths with the "false positives" spoken by Seagrave and Grisso [5]. In any case, we still have a lot of work to do on the measurement of juvenile psychopathy, without, however, invalidating the allowance for its existence.

2. Final considerations

The dissent among the experts on the main issues is a reality, so it would not be correct of us to accept this task as accomplished. The objections of some relate to matters that are substantive in substance and others with non-substantive aspects of ethical and legal relevance. In both cases, they should not be ignored. In the case of adult psychopathy, we seem to be moving toward consensus as to its existence as a clinical-forensic category distinct from the general disorders of antisocial behavior. But even there, many areas of shadow and conceptual indetermination remain. We do not yet know, for example, what is the essential nucleus of psychopathy, whether it has only one or several distinct forms, whether it is preferentially conceptualized as a taxonomic entity or as a dimensional configuration of the personality, and we ignore much about its etiology and about whether or not it has biological origin. These indeterminacies are transposed, for a majority of reasons, into their early or "incipient" manifestations, so it would be unreasonable to imagine that the investigation of psychopathy between pre-adult populations could simply be discarded from these difficulties. It can also be said that decisive progress in the field of adolescent and juvenile psychopathy will only occur when the study of adult psychopathy advances in the clarification of these fundamental subjects.

But, if this is true, it will be no less true that advances in adult psychopathy studies also depend on the research of its larval or incipient forms. As in biology, the knowledge of adult organisms benefits from what is revealed about the embryonic and growth processes, here again, it will be not only important but also *necessary* to get to know how this peculiar constellation of personality is established. Therefore, the doubts and reservations about the juvenile and adolescent psychopathy—however legitimate—must yield to the urgency and the need for research. These reserves assume, from the outset, a global character, which will consist of asking whether it is correct to speak, in a general way, of personality disorders in adolescence. We discussed this issue,

http://dx.doi.org/10.5772/intechopen.68963

possibly not as deeply as we would wish, not because it is not so important, but because the deepening would take us too far in a work of this nature, which has obvious limitations of space and ambition. We have quoted the point of view of reference specialists, as Kernberg et al. [18]., for whom it is legitimate to say, not only that there are personality disorders (PD) in adolescence, but their emergence is probably earlier, dating in many cases of early childhood. However, we need many more studies, especially of longitudinal nature, that will allow us to clarify the forms of manifestation and the degree of stability that PD can present before adulthood.

In the case of psychopathy itself, the situation is perhaps a little better than in the other personality disorders. Psychopathy is, for both intrinsic and historical reasons [61], a personality disorder *par excellence*, which has allowed, especially in the last 10 years, a number of significant advances in its incipient manifestations. However, much remains to be clarified, of course, but there is already enough information today that allows us to state, without much risk of error, that we are not investigating a mirage. We have seen that the notion of incipient psychopathy may contribute, like its adult counterpart, to clarify the clinical confusion prevailing in traditional ODD and CD categories [62, 63] We have also seen that there are instruments for measuring juvenile psychopathy—or psychopathic traits, if we prefer a less committed scientific and ethical expression—that present similar psychometric characteristics (such as PCL: YV) or, at least, sufficiently similar to the adult reference instruments (APSD and the mCPS), to the extent that they allow a quantitative rather than just clinical approach to the phenomenology in question. This approach has, for its part, sustained the establishment of a set of theoretical relations between the construct of juvenile psychopathy and other pertinent constructs and variables, which together make up a nomological network similar to that of adult psychopathy. Lynam [42] has shown that the clinical description by experts of "incipient psychopathy" can be mapped similarly to the adult version in the *Big Five* terms, and that, at least in phenomenological terms, the two constructs correspond closely. We mentioned studies of genetic heredity and laboratory tradition that show that young people and adolescents with psychopathic traits identified by these instruments exhibit deficits similar to those of their adult counterparts in many of the investigated neurofunctional dimensions.

These considerations are, in our perspective, enough to legitimize the research we have proposed. We cannot assert here adamantly that adolescent psychopathy exists as a stabilized personality disorder and that it assumes an equal (or even sufficiently similar) development to adult psychopathy.

Author details

Margarida Simões[1]* and Rui Abrunhosa Gonçalves[2]

*Address all correspondence to: margaridas@utad.pt

1 Department of Education and Psychology, University of Trás-os-Montes and Alto Douro, Quinta dos Prados, Portugal

2 School of Psychology, University of Minho, Campus de Gualtar, Braga, Portugal

References

[1] Bowlby J. Fourty-four juvenile thieves: Their characters and home life. International Journal of Psycho-Analysis. 1994;**25**:19-52

[2] Frick P, O'Brien B, Wootton J, McBurnett K. Psychopathy and conduit problems in children. Journal of Abnormal Psychology. 1994;**103**:700-707

[3] Lynam D. Early identification of chronic offenders: Who is the fledgling psychopath?. Psychological Bulletin. 1996;**120**:209-234

[4] Frick P. Juvenile psychopathy from a developmental perspective: Implications for construct development and use in forensic assessments. Law and Human Behavior. 2002;**26**(2):247-253. DOI: 10.1023/A:1014600311758

[5] Seagrave D, Grisso T. Adolescent development and the measurement of juvenile psychopathy. Law and Human Behavior. 2002;**26**:219-239. DOI: 10.1023/A:1014696110850

[6] Hart S, Watt K, Vincent G. Commentary on Seagrave and Grisso: Impressions of the state of the art. Law and Human Behavior. 2002;**26**(2):241-245

[7] Wallon H. L'enfant turbulent. Paris: Alcan, Presse Universitaires de France; 1925

[8] Bruner J. Actos de significado. Para uma psicologia cultural. Lisboa: Edições. 70; 1990

[9] Caspi A, Roberts B, Shiner R. Personality development: Stability and change. Annual Review of Psychology. 2005;**56**:453-484

[10] Caspi A, Shiner R. Personality development. In: Eisenberg N, editors. Handbook of Child Psychology: Social, Emotional, and Personality Development. Vol. 3. Hoboken, New Jersey: John Wiley & Sons; 2006. pp. 300-365

[11] Thomas A, Birch H, Chess S, Hertzig M, Korn S. Behavioral Individuality in Early Childhood. New York: New York University Press; 1963

[12] McCrae R, Costa P. A five-factor theory of personality. In: Pervin L, John O, editors. Handbook of Personality: Theory and Research.2nd ed. New York: Guilford Press; 1999. pp. 139-153

[13] Van Lieshout C, Haselager G. The big five personality factores in Q-sort descriptions of children and adolescents. In: Halverson Jr, Kohnstamm Martin R, editors. The Developing Structure of Temperament and Personality from Infancy to Adulthood. Hillsdale, NJ: Lawrence Erlbaum Associates; 1994. pp. 293-317

[14] Roberts B, DelVecchio W. The rank-order consistency of personality traits from childhood to old age: A quantitative review of longitudinal studies. Psychological Bulletin. 2000;**126**(1):3-25

[15] Roberts B, Walton K, Viechtbauer W. Patterns of mean-level change in personality traits across the life course: A meta-analysis of longitudinal studies. Psychological Bulletin. 2006;**132**(1):1-25

[16] Block J. Lives Through Time. Berkeley California: Bancroft Books; 1971

[17] American Psychiatric Association. Diagnostic and Statistical Manual of Mental Disorders. 5th Ed. Arlington: APA; 2013

[18] Kernberg P, Weiner A, Bardenstein K. Personality disorders in children and adolescents. New York: Basic Books; 2000

[19] Lynam D. Psychopathy from the perspective of the five factor model. In: Costa P, Widiger, T. editors. Personality Disorders and the Five-Factor Model of Personality. 2nd ed. Washington: American Psychological Association; 2002. pp. 325-350

[20] Bernstein D, Cohen P, Velez C, Schwab-Stone M. Prevalence and stablility of the DSM-III-R personality disorders in a community-based survey of adolescents. American Journal of Psychiatry. 1993;**150**:1237-1243

[21] Caspi A. The child is father of the man: Personality continuities from childhood to adulthood. Journal of Personality and Social Psychology. 2000;**78**(1):158-172

[22] Lynam DR. Fledgling psychopathy: A view from personality theory. Law and Human Behavior. 2002b;**26**(2):255-259. DOI: 10.1023/A:1014652328596

[23] Salekin R. Psychopathy and therapeutic pessimism: Clinical lore or clinical reality?. Clinical Psychology Review. 2002;**22**(1):79-112

[24] Harris G, Rice M. Treatment of psychopathy: A review of empirical findings. In: Patrick C, editors. Handbook of Psychopathy. New York: Guilford Press; 2006. pp. 555-572

[25] Dolan M. Psychopathic personality in young people. Advances in Psychiatric Treatment. 2004;**10**(6):466-473

[26] Kotler, McMahon. Child psychopathy: Theories, measurement, and relations with the development and persistence of conduct problems. Clinical Child and Family Psychology Review. 2005;**8**:4. DOI: 10.1007/s10567-005-8810-5

[27] Lynam D, Gudonis L. The development of psychopathy. Annual Review of Clinical Psychology. 2005;**1**:381-407

[28] Salekin R. Psychopathy in children and adolescents: Key issues in conceptualization and assessment. In: Patrick C, editors. Handbook of Psychopathy. New York: Guilford Press; 2006. pp. 389-414

[29] Klingzell l, Fanti K, Colins O, Frogner L, Andershed A, Andershed H. Early childhood trajectories of conduct problems and callous-unemotional traits: The role of fearlessness and psychopathic personality dimensions. Child Psychiatry & Human Development. 2016;**47**(2):236-247. DOI: 10.1007/s10578-015-0560-0

[30] Forsman M, Liechtenstein P, Andershed H, Larsson H. Genetic effects explain the stability of psychopathic traits from mid-to late adolescence. Journal of Abnormal Psycology. 2008;**117**:660-617.DOI: 10.1037/0021-843X.117.3.606

[31] Salekin R, Rosenbaum J, Lee Z. Child and adolescent psychopathy: Stability and change. Psychiatry, Psychology and Law. 2008;**15**(2):224-236. DOI: 10.1080/13218710802014519

[32] Frick, P. Callous-unemotional traits and conduct problems: Applying the two-factor model of psychopathy to children. In: Cooke D, Forth A, Hare R, editors. Psychopathy: Theory, Research and Implications for Society. Boston: Kluver; 1998. pp. 161-187

[33] Salekin R, Frick P. Psychopathy in children and adolescents: The need for a developmental perspective. Journal of Abnormal Child Psychology. 2005;**33**(4):403-409. DOI: 10.1007/s10802-005-5722-2

[34] Kosson D, Cyterski T, Steuerwald B, Neumann C, Walker-Matthews S. The reliability and validity of the psychopathy checklist: Youth version (PCL:YV) in non-incarcerated adolescent males. Psychological Assessment. 2002;**14**(1):97-109

[35] Salekin R, Neumann C, Leistico A, Zalot A. Psychopathy in youth and intelligence: An investigation of Cleckley's hypothesis. Journal of Clinical Child and Adolescent Psychology. 2004;**33**: 731-742

[36] Lynam, D. Pursuing the psychopath: Capturing the fledgling psychopath in a nomological net. Journal of Abnormal Psychology.1997;**106**(3):425-438

[37] Catchpole R, Gretton H. The predictive validity of risk assessment with violent young offenders: A 1-year examination of criminal outcome. Criminal Justice Behaviour. 2003;**30**:688-708

[38] Corrado R, Vincent G, Hart S, Cohen I. Predictive validity of the psychopathy checklist: Youth version for general and violent recidivism. Behavioral Sciences and the Law. 2004;**22**(1):5-22

[39] Gretton H, Hare R, Catchpole R. Psychopathy and offending from adolescence to adulthood: A 10-year follow-up. Journal of Consulting and Clinical Psychology. 2004;**72**(4):636-645

[40] Murrie D, Cornell D, Kaplan S, McConville D, Levy-Elkon A. Psychopathy Scores and violence among juvenile offenders: A multi-measure study. Behavioral Sciences and the Law. 2004;**22**(1):49-67

[41] O'Neill M, Lidz V, Heilbrun K. Adolescents with psychopathic characteristics in a substance abusing cohort: Treatment process and outcomes. Law and Human Behavior. 2003;**27**(3):299-313

[42] Lynam D, Derefinko K. Psychopathy and Personality. In: Patrick C, editors. Handbook of Psychopathy. New York: Guilford Press; 2006. pp. 133-155

[43] Lynam D. Child and adolescent psychopathy and personality. In: Salekin R, Lynam D, editors. Handbook of Child and Adolescent Psychopathy. New York: Guilford Press; 2010. pp. 179-201

[44] Costa P, McCrae R. Revised NEO Personality Inventory (NEO-PI-R) and NEO Five-Factor Inventory (NEO-FFI) Professional Manual. Odessa, FL: Psychological Assessment Resources; 1992

[45] Tellegen A, Walker N, editors. Exploring personality through test construction: Development of the multidimensional personality questionnaire. In: Briggs S, Cheeks J, editors. Personality Measures: Development and Evaluation. Vol. 1. Greenwich, CT: JAI Press; 2002. pp. 133-161

[46] Eysenck S, Eysenck H. Crime and personality: An empirical study of the three-factor theory. British Journal of Criminology. 1970;**10**:225-239

[47] Miller J, Lynam D, Widiger T, Leukefeld C. Personality disorders as extreme variants of common personality dimensions: Can the five-factor model adequately represent psychopathy?. Journal of Personality. 2001;**69**(2):253-276

[48] Cooke D, Michie C. Refining the construct of psychopathy: Towards a hierarchical model. Psychological Assessment. 2001;**13**(2):171-188

[49] Hare R, Neumann C. The PCL-R assessment of psychopathy. In Patrick C, editors. Handbook of Psychopathy. New York: Guilford Press; 2006. pp. 58-88

[50] Cooke D, Michie C, Hart S. (2006). Facets of clinical psychopathy. In Patrick C. editors. Handbook of Psychopathy New York: Guilford Press; 2006. pp. 91-106

[51] Irún M. Validez del modelo de las cuatro facetas de la psicopatia de R. D. Hare (2003) en una muestra penitenciaria: evidencia desde el laboratorio psicofisiológico. [thesis]. Catellón: Universitat Jaume I; 2007

[52] Forth A, Kosson D, Hare R. The Psychopathy checklist: Youth version. Toronto, Canada: Multi-Health Systems. 2003

[53] Odgers C, Reppucci N, Moretti M. Nipping psychopathy in the bud: An examination of the convergent, predictive, and theoretical utility of the PCL-YV among adolescent girls. Behavioral Sciences and the Law. 2005;**23**(6):743-763

[54] Salekin R, Brannen D, Zalot A, Leistico A, Neumann C. Factor structure of psychopathy in youth: Testing the applicability of the new four-factor model. Criminal Justice and Behavior. 2006;**33**(2):135-157

[55] Vitacco M, Neumann C, Caldwell M, Leistico A, Van Rybroek G. Testing factor models of the psychopathy checklist: Youth version and their association with instrumental aggression. Journal of Personality Assessment. 2006;**87**(1):74-83

[56] Jackson R, Rogers R, Neumann C, Lambert P. Psychopathy in female offenders: An investigation of its underlying dimensions. Criminal Justice and Behavior. 2002;**29**(6):692-704. DOI: 10.1177/0306624X16648109

[57] Frick P, Hare R. Antisocial Process Screening Device. Toronto, Canada: Multi-Health Systems; 2001

[58] Frick P, Bodin S, Barry C. Psychopathic traits and conduct problems in community and clinic-referred samples of children: Further development of the psychopathy screening device. Psychological Assessment. 2000; **12**(4):382-393

[59] Vitacco M, Rogers R, Neumann C. The antisocial process screening device: An examination of its construct and criterion-related validity. Assessment. 2003;**10**(2):143-150

[60] Lynam D, Caspi A, Moffitt T, Raine A, Loeber R, Stouthamer-Loeber M. Adolescent psychopathy and the big five: Results from two samples. Journal of Abnormal Child Psychology. 2005;**33**(4):431-443

[61] Blackburn R. Personality disorder and psychopathy: Conceptual and empirical integration. Psychology, Crime and Law. 2007;**13**(1):7-18

[62] Moffit T. Adolescence limited and life-course–persistent anti-social behavior: A developmental taxonomy. Psychological Review. 1993;**4**:674-701

[63] Moffitt T. Life—course-persistent versus adolescent-limited antisocial behavior. In: Cicchetti D, Cohen D, editors. Developmental Psychopathology (Volume 3): Risk, Disorder, and Adaptation. 2nd. ed. Hoboken: John Wiley & Sons; 2006. pp. 570-578

The Relationship between Emotional Distress and Cognitive Coping Strategies in Adolescents with Conduct Disorder (CD)

Roxana Șipoș and Elena Predescu

Additional information is available at the end of the chapter

http://dx.doi.org/10.5772/intechopen.70817

Abstract

Conduct disorder (CD) is a matter of societal concern because of the significant burden for the patient, family and immediate environment and the strong associations with school failure, disrupted peer and family relationships, excessive risk-taking and addictive behaviors. The economic costs of aggressive and antisocial behavior in children and adolescents are huge. The mechanisms that lead individuals to adopt such behaviors have been defined and approached from various perspectives. Our purpose was to assess the emotional distress, irrational beliefs, emotion regulation strategies and callousness, uncaring, unemotional traits in a sample of adolescents diagnosed with conduct disorder and to investigate the relationship between them. The adolescents with conduct disorder had a low level of emotional distress and negative dysfunctional emotions. Girls reported a higher level of emotional distress than boys and significantly lower positive emotions. We found significant correlations between the emotional distress reported by the adolescents and their irrational cognitions. The suppression and reassessment strategies did not register values above those of the general population. No significant relation was found between emotional distress and the emotional regulation strategies reappraisal and suppression. The use of suppression related significantly with callousness, uncaring, and unemotional traits. The reappraisal coping strategy related significantly only with uncaring trait, the relation being negative. Research findings from different areas correlated with pathology may improve current therapies (i.e., including emotion regulation training in individualized intervention protocol) or help to develop new ones.

Keywords: emotional distress, emotion regulation, irrational beliefs, callous/unemotional traits, conduct disorder, adolescents

1. Introduction

Conduct disorder (CD) is one of the main diagnosis for which consultations are required in specialized mental health services for children and adolescents. Polanczyk et al. published in 2015, a meta-analysis of 41 studies conducted between 1985 and 2012 in 27 countries. They estimated that the prevalence of mental disorders in children and adolescents worldwide is 13.4% (approximately 241 million young people around the world are affected by a mental disorder). The most common categories identified were disruptive disorders with a prevalence of 5.7% (affecting 113 million children), oppositional defiant disorder (ODD) 3.6%, and CD 2.1% [1]. Canino et al. included 25 studies in a meta-regression for CD and ODD, and the results showed a prevalence of CD estimated at 3.2%, with no significant variability on estimates of CD and ODD from studies conducted in North America and Europe [2]. The economic costs of aggressive and antisocial behavior in children and adolescents are huge. Romeo et al. in their sample of referred children (representing about a quarter of all cases of CD), reported the average annual total cost of £5960, but the largest cost burden of £4637, was borne by the family [3]. In 2012, Olesen et al. estimated that in Europe, 2.1 million subjects are affected by CD with direct health costs of 352 billion euros and direct non-medical costs of 3319 billion euros [4]. Thus, the importance of accurate and early identification of CD is supported by long-term implications on child and family functioning [5]. These often extend to the academic, social, and interpersonal relationships with peers or adults. Consequently, prompt access of children, adolescents, and family members to specialized services would avoid unnecessary and costly complications. The required interventions should be personalized, comprising the cognitive and emotional profile of the child and delivered timely. This way, the costs with lifetime care for each person may be reduced, through the effects on quality of life and well-being.

1.1. Definitions, actual classification

Both of the psychiatric classification systems used in clinical practice worldwide (ICD-10 and DSM-V) describe the essential features of CD as a repetitive and persistent pattern of behavior through which the basic rights of others or major age-appropriate societal norms or rules are repeatedly violated beginning in childhood or adolescence [6, 7]. DSM-V defines CDs based on 15 behavioral criteria that can be categorized into four generalized behavioral subtypes: (1) aggression to people and animals, (2) destruction of property, (3) deceitfulness or theft, and (4) serious violations of rules. Another mandatory requirement is that the disturbance in behavior causes clinically significant impairment in social, academic or occupational functioning [6]. Also, the DSM-V makes possible the distinction between childhood and adolescent-onset forms of CD. The WHO's ICD-10 divides the CD into socialized conduct disorder, unsocialized conduct disorder (to highlight the significant problems in developing peer relationships), conduct disorder confined to the family context, and ODD [7]. One of the major changes in DSM-V is the addition of psychopathic callous-unemotional (CU) traits as a new specifier. This entity is indicated as "with limited prosocial emotions." The concept includes the lack of remorse and empathy, lack of concern about school performance, and the manipulative

http://dx.doi.org/10.5772/intechopen.70817

use of emotional display for personal gain. Consistent with the affective dimension of adult psychopathy, CU traits also include a lack of concern for others feelings and shallow affects.

1.2. Callous-unemotional traits and conduct disorder

Moffitt's development taxonomy describes two primary types of offenders, short-term adolescent offenders and life-course-persistent offenders [8]. This is one of the most recognized and persistent subtyping schemes of CD based on longitudinal research, indicating that youth with CD onset in childhood are at higher risk for exhibiting persistent criminal behavior into adulthood [9]. Moffitt's theory has made remarkable contributions to practice, including the possibility of identifying children at risk, but it did not integrate the elements of psychopathy concept with emotional and cognitive differences that can predict the disorder severity and risks. Another central theory in the field is that of Frick who considers focusing on the person's affective and interpersonal style to designate subgroups of antisocial individuals which is the hallmark of the psychopathy construct [10]. Consequently, it is possible to identify a subgroup of children with childhood-onset CD presenting callous-unemotional (CU) features [10].

In terms of prevalence, Kahn et al. reported that in a community sample, 10–32% of those with CD and 2–7% of those without CD met the callous-unemotional (CU) specifier and in a clinic-referred sample, 21–50% of those with CD and 14–32% of those without CD met the CU specifier [11]. Rowe reported similar result, 2.9% of the pediatric population had high CU traits, while only less than one-third of them also met the criteria for CD [12]. CU traits may appear outside the CD diagnosis, and another important research direction is set by the investigation of CU traits outside the CD diagnosis [13]. Children with CU traits show more behavioral problems, more severe aggression, and more proactive aggression than other children with CD [14]. Current studies describe high CU traits prevalence in youth with CD ranging from 10 to 46% in community samples to 21–59% in clinical samples [11, 12]. Forward longitudinal studies are needed on the consequences of having high, intermediate, and low levels of CU traits among children who meet the criteria for CD [15].

Most studies indicate that youth with elevated CU traits are at risk of developing severe and persistent antisocial behavior. Those with CD and the CU specifier showed higher rates of aggression in both community and clinic-referred samples, and higher cruelty rates in the clinic-referred samples [11]. The adolescent offenders with CD and the CU specifier showed more severe antisocial acts, delinquency, and higher recidivism rates [10, 16]. In longitudinal studies, CU traits emerged beside depression and drug use as the strongest predictors of later antisocial behavior [17]. The available studies indicate that CU traits have a stable characteristic that predicts poor outcome and suggests the hypothesis, not yet tested, that these traits represent the childhood-onset life-course persistent CD subtype.

1.3. Callous-unemotional traits, conduct disorder, and internalizing symptoms

Children and adolescents with CD with and without CU traits differ in their emotional, cognitive, and personality profiles. Although comorbidity rates are higher with other externalizing disorders (i.e., ADHD-Attention-deficit/hyperactivity disorder or ODD-oppositional defiant disorder), there is also important overlap with internalizing disorders (i.e., depression and anxiety) [15, 18]. One longitudinal study found that increase in conduct disorder symptoms and CU traits was accompanied by increase in anxiety, depressive symptoms, narcissism, proactive and reactive aggression and decrease in self-esteem [19]. Other studies reported that chldren with high conduct problems alone were characterized by anxiety and increased physiological reactions to emotional stimuli compared to those with high CU traits and normal controls [20], contrary to anterior results [21]. Regarding the association between anxiety, depression, and the CU traits, research results are generally inconsistent [21]. Kahn explained the relation between high CU traits and anxiety, manifested by higher levels of impulsivity, externalizing behaviors, aggression, and behavioral activation, through a history of abuse [22].

CU traits in antisocial youth have been associated with deficits in emotionally distressing stimuli processing in numerous studies. A different pattern of emotional reactivity may characterize distinct subgroups of youth with antisocial behavior problems [23]. Children with CU traits and conduct problems seem less reactive to threatening and emotionally distressing stimuli than other antisocial youth using a number of different methods [10]. Different emotional profiles and emotional regulation processes may contribute to the development and expression of reactive and instrumental aggression [24]. Children that rated high in instrumental aggression were less emotionally reactive than those rated low in instrumental aggression [25]. Also, the associations between aggression, psychopathic traits, and responsiveness to distressing stimuli did not differ for boys and girls [26]. Similar results were reported by Muñoz et al. in a study on 85 adolescent boys placed in a juvenile detention center [27]. Sharp showed that the CU traits are associated with deficits in recognizing emotions over and above other psychopathy dimensions, and this relationship is driven by a specific deficit in recognizing complex emotions more so than basic emotions [28]. Most of the studies have generally shown that CU traits are related to a deficit in the child's affective experience of empathic concern to the distress of others. Current evidences support the low level of internalization problems in those with CD and high CU traits, in terms of both dysfunctional emotions and total emotional distress.

1.4. Callous-unemotional traits, conduct disorder, and cognitive emotion regulation strategies

Attempts to identify and classify emotional regulation strategies have led in time to the development of more paradigms [29, 30]. In relation to psychological pathology, emotional regulation strategies have been approached from an adaptive (i.e., reassessment, acceptance) or maladaptive (i.e., suppression, rumination) point of view. It is, however, considered that the psychological disorder is rather the result of their inflexible use. In most studies, maladaptive emotional regulation strategies are described as associated with aggressive behaviors. The adolescents' difficulty in regulating anger or depression negative emotions has been associated with their use of physical and relational aggression [31]. There is evidence that inflexible use of avoidance and suppression strategies can lead to aggressive behavior [32, 33] or can predict aggressive behavior even after anger control [34]. Instead, reassessment is more effective in reducing anger than attempts to suppress or accept it [35].

Children with CU traits show a decreased level of emotion problems and, consequently, cognitive emotion regulation strategies seem to be more important for children without CU. Deficits in emotion regulation strategies directly (i.e., acting aggressively due to intense anger) or indirectly (i.e., by making the child more difficult to discipline) lead to the development of conduct problems [10]. Children with anger regulation problems often exhibit early oppositional/defiant behaviors, which tend to precede the development of CD in childhood [36].

1.5. Callous-unemotional traits, conduct disorder and cognitive behavioral therapy (CBT) interventions

CU traits may also be important when implementing treatment for CD children. Treatment options include parenting interventions and multisystemic therapy [37]. The therapeutic interventions possibilities are relatively limited and among those with proven efficacy are cognitive behavioral approaches. In REBT psychopathological model, primary and secondary irrational beliefs (maladaptive and hot cognitions) determine dysfunctional (positive or negative) emotions that translate into signs/symptoms at cognitive, emotional, behavioral and physiological level [38, 39]. Consequently, it is necessary to do a cognitive and emotional profile as complete as possible in order to choose and customize the most appropriate form of intervention. One of the most important irrational beliefs is low frustration tolerance which means that one cannot bear certain circumstances making a situation intolerable. The link between the irrational beliefs (frustration intolerance toward norms, work; demands for fairness) and anger negative dysfunctional emotion was demonstrated in several studies. In Fives's study, male gender, anger, and the irrational belief frustration intolerance to norms predicted aggression, but the combination between anger and frustration intolerance to norms was a better predictor for physical aggression [40].

Children with CU traits did not show improvements after punishment-oriented behavior modification programs [41] or are less responsive to typical parental socialization practices than other children with conduct problems [42]. An explanation for these poor outcomes may be the fact that children with CD and high level of CU traits are less distressed by the effect of their behavior on others [43]. Also, response to behavioral treatment seems to be poor and often needs booster sessions to maintain the improvements [44]. Buitelar considers that one of the greatest challenges is to develop, test, and implement new effective treatments for CD children with high levels of CU traits [45]. CU traits should be studied in relation with the response to existing CD treatments.

However, there are not enough studies to explain clearly the mechanism by which cognitive components such as irrational beliefs lead to the appearance of dysfunctional negative emotions—anger type and subsequently to the emergence of aggressive behaviors. In principle, emotional regulation cognitive strategies (i.e., reappraisal or suppression) can influence the level of emotional distress and, consequently, the behavioral reactions.

Our main objective was to assess the emotional distress, irrational beliefs, emotion regulation strategies and callousness, uncaring, unemotional traits in a sample of adolescents diagnosed with conduct disorder. Secondary, we wanted to investigate the relationship between emotional distress, irrational cognitions, emotional regulation strategies and callous/unemotional traits and the effects of irrational beliefs and emotion regulation strategies on distress. We conducted a cross-sectional clinical trial on a sample of adolescents diagnosed with conduct disorder.

2. Method

2.1. Participants

Data comes from 60 adolescents aged 14–18 years with a diagnosis of conduct disorder according to international diagnosis criteria Diagnostic and Statistical Manual of Mental Disorders, Fourth Edition, Text Revision (DSM IV-TR) (DSM IV-TR was used because the Diagnostic and Statistical Manual of Mental Disorders, Fifth Edition (DSM-5) was not available in Romanian at that time), who reported verbal or physical aggressive acts. The adolescents included in the study were patients in the Child and Adolescent Psychiatry Clinic from Cluj-Napoca, Romania between January 2015 and July 2015. Children diagnosed and treated in this clinic come from all the country and are diverse in terms of socioeconomic status.

We included in the study: boys or girls aged 14–18 with diagnosis of conduct disorder according to DSM IV-TR international criteria; QI > 80; agreement (adolescent and caregiver) to participate to the study after the purpose and protocol of the study were explained.

We excluded from the study: adolescents with known severe medical conditions; major accidents or stressors in the last 6 months; diagnosis of learning disorders (dyslexia); diagnosis of psychotic disorders; diagnosis of autism spectrum disorder; QI < 80; adolescents placed in foster care or institutionalized.

2.2. Instruments

For the diagnostic procedure, we used the Structured Clinical Interview for DSM-IV Childhood Disorders (Kid-SCID), which is a semi-structured interview for child and adolescent classification of psychiatric disorders. To assess the intellectual coefficient, we used the Raven's Progressive Matrices.

To assess emotions and the level of distress, we used Profile of Affective Distress (PAD)—a rating scale with 39 items that assesses subjective dimensions of positive and negative emotions (functional and dysfunctional) [46].

To assess the irrational beliefs, we used the General Attitudes and Beliefs Scale-Short Version (GABS-SV) [48], a self-report instrument with 26-items grouped into 8 specific subscales, that measures the irrational beliefs [47–50]: the need for achievement, the need for approval, the need for comfort, demands for fairness, self-downing, other-downing, rationality and irrational beliefs. GABS-SV allows the measuring of a global score for irrational beliefs as a result of the first six dimensions above. GABS-SV is based on current REBT theory, in which people who formulate their wishes in terms of imperative needs, have a high potential for generating emotional stress [38, 51–53].

To evaluate emotional regulation strategies, we used the Emotion Regulation Questionnaire (ERQ)—a 10 items scale (6 items measures the frequency of using reappraisal as an emotional regulation method and 4 items measures the frequency of suppression use). ERQ was developed by Gross and John [30] to measure the usual, habitual, reappraisal, and suppression use. Respondents choose a score for each item on a 7-point Likert scale ranging from 1 (strong disagreement) to 7 (strong agreement). Also, the authors ask for the order of items not to be reversed during the scale administration. The published results indicate that ERQ is a valid tool to measure individual differences in suppression and reappraisal. The scale is translated and adapted in many languages (www.spl.stanford.edu/resources.htlm) and has acceptable internal consistency indicators.

The Inventory of Callous-Unemotional Traits (ICU) is a 24-item questionnaire designed for the comprehensive assessment of insensitivity, lack of remorse and concern for others, callous/unemotional traits. These features proved to be important for the description of a distinct group of teenagers with antisocial and aggressive behaviors. The questionnaire has three subscales: callousness, uncaring, and unemotional. Item scoring is done on a Likert scale of 4 points from 0 (not true) to 3 (definitely true). The instrument can be applied to children aged 13–17 years [54, 55]. All psychometric instruments used are specific and standardized.

2.3. Design

Adolescents who agreed to participate in the study received additional information and signed informed consent. Psychiatric and somatic assessments were performed in order to determine eligibility, confirm the diagnosis and detect the possible co-morbidities. Each adolescent was psychologically assessed in order to determine the developmental level. The psychiatric examination comprised anamnesis, psychiatric evaluation, clinical observation and parental interview, including the Kid-SCID semi-structured clinical interview for infant, child, and adolescent disorders. The participants met the international diagnostic criteria DSM IV-TR for conduct disorder. Medical data have been supplemented with those in patients' observation charts and medical records.

After the clinical interview, the somatic exam, and psychological assessment, the adolescents filled in the assessment scales for emotions and the level of distress, irrational beliefs, emotional regulation strategies, and callous/unemotional features. The questionnaires were analyzed according to the instructions specified by the authors in the user manual. The participants filled in the questionnaire individually, without time limit.

2.4. Data analysis

The statistical software used for data analysis was the SPSS 17. To describe and assess the studied population and PDA, GABS-SV, ERQ, and ICU scores, we used univariate statistical analysis (mean, median, standard deviation, and frequencies). Bivariate statistical analysis (correlation and t test) was used to identify significant associations between the emotional distress, irrational cognitions, emotional regulation strategies and the features frequently described as associated with aggressive behavior (lack of empathy, remorse, diminished emotional response) or sex differences in the studied sample.

2.5. Ethical aspects

The study was conducted in compliance with international ethical standards setout in the Helsinki Declaration of Human Rights updated. All the adolescents included in the study signed the informed consent. Data were used ensuring the privacy and subject's identity protection.

3. Results

Sixty patients with ages between 14 and 18 years, with psychiatric diagnosis of conduct disorder and aggressive behaviors were included in the study. Of the 60 patients' enrolled, 22 were girls and 38 were boys. The sex ratio (male: female) was 1.72:1. Mean age of patients was M = 16.16 years (SD = 1.25), with M = 15.90 years (SD = 1.19) for girls and M = 16.31 years (SD = 1.27) for boys.

3.1. Distress scores

The assessment of the subjective dimension of the negative and positive, and functional and dysfunctional emotions, reported by the PAD questionnaire, indicates a low overall emotional distress mean score compared with the Romanian general population norms M = 32.46 (SD = 20.63) and would characterize this sample as having a low negative emotions. On all the other domains measured by PAD, negative functional emotions (sadness, worry) and negative dysfunctional emotions (depression, anxiety), adolescents with conduct disorder scored lower than the Romanian general population norms (see **Table 1**). Girls reported a higher level of overall emotional distress score M = 38.36 SD = 18.65 (the upper limit of the class II—low level of emotional distress) when compared to boys M = 29.05 SD = 21.19 (the lower limit of class II level of emotional distress).

Analyses performed separately for the two sex categories revealed statistically significant differences for negative dysfunctional emotion depression ($t(58) = -2.79$, $p = 0.007$) and positive emotions ($t(58) = 4.15$, $p < 0.05$), the girls scoring significantly higher on negative dysfunctional emotion depression than the boys and significantly lower on positive emotions, but still lower than the general population means.

3.2. Irrationality scores

The assessment of irrational cognitions with GABS-SV has highlighted medium level of irrationality for the studied sample. The adolescents scored on the medium level for all the dimensions measured by GABS-SV (the need for achievement, the need for approval, the need for comfort, demands for fairness, self-downing, other-downing, rationality, and irrational beliefs),

	Sex	N	Mean	Std. Deviation	Std. Error Mean
PAD					
Emotional distress total score	Boys	38	29.05	21.19	3.43
	Girls	22	38.36	18.65	3.97
	Total	60	32.46	20.63	2.66
Negative dysfunctional emotions depression	Boys	38	6.84	6.72	1.09
	Girls	22	11.90	6.82	1.45
	Total	60	8.7	7.14	0.92
Negative dysfunctional emotions anxiety	Boys	38	6.15	4.87	0.791
	Girls	22	8.63	5.62	1.19
	Total	60	7.06	5.25	0.67
Positive emotions	Boys	38	30.05	9.88	1.60
	Girls	22	19.63	8.32	1.77
	Total	60	26.23	10.56	1.36
GABS SV					
Need for achievement	Boys	38	11.36	3.24	0.52
	Girls	22	13.27	1.16	0.24
	Total	60	12.06	2.81	0.36
Need for approval	Boys	38	8.42	2.26	0.36
	Girls	22	9.81	2.34	0.49
	Total	60	8.93	2.37	0.30
Need for comfort	Boys	38	11.31	2.52	0.40
	Girls	22	13.36	1.25	0.26
	Total	60	12.06	2.35	0.30
Demands for fairness	Boys	38	12.63	2.63	0.42
	Girls	22	14.45	2.19	0.46
	Total	60	13.30	2.61	0.33
Self-downing	Boys	38	10.21	2.78	0.45
	Girls	22	12.00	2.35	0.50
	Total	60	10.86	2.75	0.35
Other-downing	Boys	38	8.36	2.35	0.38
	Girls	22	9.63	2.10	0.44
	Total	60	8.83	2.33	0.30

	Sex	N	Mean	Std. Deviation	Std. Error Mean
Rationality	Boys	38	14.73	2.68	0.43
	Girls	22	14.54	2.66	0.56
	Total	60	14.66	2.65	0.34
Irrational beliefs	Boys	38	62.31	9.30	1.50
	Girls	22	72.54	5.90	1.25
	Total	60	66.06	9.56	1.23
ERQ					
Suppression	Boys	38	12.78	3.18	0.51
	Girls	22	12.81	3.17	0.67
	Total	60	12.80	3.15	0.40
Reappraisal	Boys	38	19.10	3.87	0.62
	Girls	22	20.18	2.61	0.55
	Total	60	19.50	3.48	0.44
ICU					
ICU callousness	Boys	38	10.94	5.64	0.91
	Girls	22	8.27	5.40	1.15
	Total	60	9.96	5.65	0.73
ICU uncaring	Boys	38	10.42	5.66	0.91
	Girls	22	10.54	4.07	0.86
	Total	60	10.46	5.10	0.65
ICU unemotional	Boys	38	7.31	3.05	0.49
	Girls	22	7.54	2.10	0.44
	Total	60	7.40	2.72	0.35
ICU total score	Boys	38	28.68	11.85	1.92
	Girls	22	26.36	10.07	2.14
	Total	60	27.83	11.20	1.44

Table 1. Central tendency and dispersion indicators PAD, GABS SV, ERQ and ICU scores.

when compared with the norms for the Romanian general population (see **Table 1**). When looking separately on the two sexes, there are some differences. Boys reported a medium level of irrationality (M = 62.31, SD = 9.30), a low level on demands for fairness (M = 12.63, SD = 2.63) and a medium level on self-downing (M = 10.21, SD = 2.78), while girls reported a high level of irrationality (M = 72.54, SD = 5.90), a medium level on demands for fairness (M = 14.45, SD = 2.19) and a high level on self-downing (M = 12, SD = 2.35). Analyses performed separately for the two sex categories revealed statistically significant differences for all measured dimensions (need for achievement—$t(58) = -2.65$, $p < 0.05$; need for approval—$t(58) = -2.27$, $p < 0.05$; need for comfort—$t(58) = -3.54$, $p < 0.01$; demands for fairness—$t(58) = -2.73$, $p < 0.05$; self-downing—$t(58) = -2.53$, $p < 0.05$; other-downing—$t(58) = -2.08$, $p < 0.05$; irrational beliefs—$t(58) = -4.63$, $p < 0.01$), except rationality, the girls having significantly higher irrationality scores.

3.3. Coping mechanism scores

Suppression and reappraisal coping mechanisms are used by both girls and boys with similar frequency (see **Table 1**). The means calculated for the suppressing strategy ($M = 12.8$, $SD = 3.15$) have values lower than the means for the general population. Reappraisal strategy ($M = 19.5$, $SD = 3.48$) is also less used by the adolescents in the studied group. The norms are different for males and females and the girls from our sample use these strategies less than the boys.

3.4. Insensitivity, lack of remorse/concern for others, and callous/unemotional traits

ICU measures three behavioral dimensions: callousness, uncaring, and unemotional. The callousness includes factors such as lack of empathy, guilt, and remorse for misdoings. The study sample recorded higher scores on this domain than those of the general population ($M = 9.96$, $SD = 5.65$). Boys had higher scores than the girls, but the difference did not reach the statistical significance threshold ($t(58) = 1.79$, $p = 0.07$). The uncaring factor includes a lack of caring about performance in tasks and the feelings of others. On this domain, the adolescents with conduct disorder scored also higher than the general population norms ($M = 10.46$, $SD = 5.1$), with no sex difference. The third dimension focuses on the absence of emotional expression. In this domain, the studied sample scored higher than the general population ($M = 7.4$, $SD = 2.72$), with no sex differences (see **Table 1**).

3.5. The relationship between the emotional distress, dysfunctional negative emotions (depression, anxiety), irrational beliefs and coping strategies

Assuming that the emotional distress is generated among other factors, by the child cognitive individualities, we investigated whether in this population (adolescents diagnosed with conduct disorder), the potential mediators (irrational beliefs and coping strategies) relate statistically significant to the reported emotional distress.

We analyzed the relationship between the emotional distress, negative dysfunctional emotion depression and anxiety and irrational beliefs. For all three dimensions evaluated with the PDA subscales, we obtained statistically significant and positive correlations with the irrationality score, the intensity varying from medium to high. The relationship is positive, meaning that when the level of irrationality increases, the emotional distress increases also. In terms of explanatory value, irrationality explains between 16% ($R^2 = 0.16$ for negative dysfunctional emotions anxiety score) and 31% ($R^2 = 0.31$ for negative dysfunctional emotions depression score) of the emotional distress variance. Irrationality related significantly with the level of positive emotions, the relation being negative. The irrationality dimensions that correlated with emotional distress scores were the need for achievement, the need for approval, the need for comfort, and demands for fairness. The self-downing dimension correlated only with the negative dysfunctional emotions depression scores. The relation was positive meaning that when the level of self-downing increases, the negative dysfunctional emotions depression also increases.

The suppression and reappraisal coping strategies measured by ERQ did not correlate statistically significant with PAD emotional distress scores (see **Table 2**).

3.6. The relation between the insensitivity, lack of remorse, callous traits, the irrational beliefs, and coping strategies

Because the insensitivity, lack of remorse, and callous/unemotional traits are considered to be important factors in describing a specific category of children and adolescents with conduct disorder and antisocial and aggressive behaviors, we investigated whether the irrational beliefs and coping strategies relate statistically significant to these traits measured by ICU.

As seen in **Table 3**, ICU callousness is related significantly only with the need for comfort irrationality subscale and ICU uncaring with the self-downing irrationality subscale. The relations were positive.

The suppression coping strategy (measured by ERQ) related statistically significant to all the domains measured by ICU, with intensities varying from medium to high. The determination

	Emotional distress total score	Negative dysfunctional emotions depression	Negative dysfunctional emotions anxiety	Positive emotions
Need for achievement	0.41**	0.38**	−0.33**	−0.22
Need for approval	0.38**	0.34**	−0.41**	−0.52**
Need for comfort	0.29*	0.33**	−0.26*	−0.21
Demands for fairness	0.47**	0.48**	−0.40**	−0.46**
Self-downing	0.24	0.40**	0.19	−0.11
Other-downing	−0.00	0.13	−0.11	−0.16
Rationality	−0.08	−0.22	−0.03	−0.19
Irrational beliefs	0.48**	0.56**	0.40**	−0.44**
ERQ Suppression	−0.12	−0.01	−0.06	0.06
ERQ Reappraisal	−0.18	−0.17	−0.04	0.02

*Correlations significant at $p < 0.05$;
**Correlation significant at $p < 0.01$.

Table 2. The correlation of PAD emotional distress scores with the irrational beliefs, and use of suppression/reappraisal coping strategies.

	ICU callousness	ICU uncaring	ICU unemotional	ICU total score
Need for achievement	−0.11	−0.01	0.04	−0.05
Need for approval	0.00	0.04	0.17	0.06
Need for comfort	0.29*	0.12	−0.20	−0.16
Demands for fairness	−0.16	−0.08	−0.07	−0.14
Self-downing	0.18	0.30*	0.07	0.25
Other-downing	−0.07	−0.16	−0.08	−0.13
Rationality	−0.24	−0.10	−0.09	−0.19
Irrational beliefs	−0.12	0.06	−0.01	−0.03
ERQ Suppression	0.38**	0.27*	0.41**	0.42**
ERQ Reappraisal	−0.18	−0.30*	−0.20	−0.28*

*Correlations significant at $p < 0.05$;
**Correlation significant at $p < 0.01$.

Table 3. The correlation of ICU scores with the irrational beliefs, and the use of suppression/reappraisal coping strategies.

coefficients obtained from the square of the correlation coefficients indicate that suppression explains between 7% ($R^2 = 0.07$ for ICU uncaring) and 17% ($R^2 = 0.17$ for ICU total score) of the ICU scores variance.

The reappraisal coping strategy is related significantly only with ICU uncaring and ICU total score, the relations being negative, meaning that the more frequently used is the reappraisal coping strategy the lower will be the scores at ICU.

4. Discussion

4.1. Main findings

Several studies reported that children and adolescents with conduct problems experience emotion more intensely, have difficulties in matching emotions to social cues, are more likely to feel angry in specific trigger anger situations, do not recognize their own feelings, and tend to focus on the negative aspects of situations [56, 57]. Often girls and boys at risk for conduct disorders and aggression have difficulties regulating their emotions. Children and adolescents at risk for externalizing problems have more negative emotions, less regulated emotions, and less regulated behaviors [58]. In our study, the adolescents with conduct disorder reported a low level of emotional distress and negative dysfunctional emotions (depression, anxiety) confirming the lack of a relationship between the symptoms of internalization and those of externalization with acts of aggression. Girls reported a higher level of emotional distress than boys, especially on negative dysfunctional emotion depression and significantly lower positive emotions. In a study regarding the gender differences in cognitive vulnerability to depression and behavior problems in adolescents, the cognitive variables that best explained gender differences in depressive symptoms were negative orientation toward social problems, self-focused negative cognitions, lower levels of positive automatic thoughts, the need for approval and success, the need for acceptance beliefs and other-focused negative cognitions [59].

The adolescents with conduct disorder from the studied sample scored on the medium level for all the dimensions of irrationality were measured by GABS-SV (the need for achievement, the need for approval, the need for comfort, demands for fairness, self-downing, other-downing, rationality, and irrational beliefs). Girls reported a high level of irrationality and self-downing. Analyses performed separately for the two sex categories revealed statistically significant differences for all irrationality dimensions, girls having significantly higher irrationality scores than boys. The results confirm the findings from the study regarding the gender differences in cognitive vulnerability [59]. Also, irrationality related statistically significant with all emotional distress subscales, the intensity varying from medium to high, irrationality explaining between 16 and 31% of the emotional distress variance. The irrationality dimensions that correlated with emotional distress scores were the need for achievement, the need for approval, the need for comfort, and demands for fairness. The self-downing dimension correlated only with the negative dysfunctional emotions depression scores.

Non-adaptive emotional regulation strategies are described as associated with various aggressive behaviors. The difficulty in regulating negative emotions like anger or depression has been associated with the use of physical and relational aggression in adolescents [31]. A person can override emotion by suppression. Expressive suppression occurs when a person actively tries to inhibit ongoing behavior [60]. There is evidence in the literature suggesting that inflexible use of both avoidance and suppression strategies can lead to aggressive behavior. Another study found that the use of avoidance and suppression predicts aggressive behavior, even after anger control [34].

Two emotional regulation strategies: cognitive reappraisal and acceptance have been associated with important therapeutic approaches. Reappraisal is recognized as one of the active ingredients of traditional CBT [61], while acceptance is considered central to acceptance and commitment therapy [62], dialectical behavioral therapy [63] or mindfulness therapies [64]. In an experimental study, Szasz et al. showed that reappraisal is more effective in reducing anger than suppression or acceptance of it. Moreover, the participants in reappraisal group persisted significantly longer in a frustrating task than those trained to suppress or accept negative emotions [35]. Sullivan et al. found that the difficulty of managing and coping with anger was associated with increased physical aggression among those boys who generally do not inhibit emotional expression [31].

Three emotional regulation strategies have been found in studies to be protective for the emergence of psychopathology: reappraisal, problem-solving, and acceptance. Suppression (emotions and thoughts), avoidance (experiential and behavioral), and rumination are considered risk factors. Emotional expression is less studied in the clinical population. Age moderates the relationship between psychopathology and some non-adaptive emotional regulation strategies (i.e., suppression). Children are less able to use them due to the lack of acquisition of executive control over emotional reactions [65] or difficulty in using metacognition [66, 67]. Suppression and reappraisal coping mechanisms are used by both girls and boys in the studied group, with similar frequency, but less than general population. The norms are different for males and females, and girls use these strategies less than boys.

The adolescents with behavioral disorders characterized by increased aggression, cognitive problems, and marked impulsivity, have an early onset of the disorder and a negative prognosis. A proportion of children and adolescents with conduct disorder have psychopathic traits consisting in two types of impairment: callous-unemotional traits associated with reduced empathic response to the distress of other individuals that reflects reduced amygdala responsiveness to distress cues and an impulsive-antisocial component with deficits in decision-making and reinforcement learning [68]. The Inventory of Callous-Unemotional Traits (ICU) [69] is designed for a comprehensive assessment of aggressive features, lack of empathy, lack of remorse, and reduced emotional expressivity. These features are considered to play an important role in highlighting antisocial and aggressive behaviors among adolescents.

ICU measures three behavioral dimensions: callousness, uncaring, and unemotional. The study sample recorded higher scores on all ICU domains than the general population. Boys had higher scores on callousness than the girls, but the difference did not reach the statistical significance threshold. For uncaring and unemotional domains, there were no sex differences. In recent studies, male adolescents did not report more aggressive behavior than females suggesting an increase in aggression and violence among girls [70].

Appropriate emotional regulation is a critical component for optimal child function, but there are differences in the use of emotional regulation strategies depending on the developmental level and the presence of a clinical disorder. Failure to acquire adapted emotional regulation skills leads to difficulties in social and school skills [71]. The use of suppression coping strategy, related statistically significant with all domains measured by ICU, the intensity varying from medium to high. The use of suppression explaining between 7 and 17% of the ICU scores variance. The use of reappraisal coping strategy related significantly only with ICU uncaring and ICU total score, the relations being negative. Emotion regulation using avoidance and suppression may increase aggression by exaggerating negative emotions, reducing aggression inhibition, compromising decision-making, diminishing social networks, increasing physical excitement, and preventing solving difficult situations [33].

4.2. Study limits

The study is cross-sectional and a causal relationship between the studied variables cannot be deducted. The clinical sample size was relatively small. The instruments were filled in by the adolescents and the answers reflect their perception on the measures proposed. Although the adolescents themselves may be the best source of information about their thoughts and emotions, for some instruments, like ICU, other respondents may offer more reliable information. The participants were asked to answer the questions considering different periods of time and the reporting accuracy could be reduced. The psychometric instruments used assessed only some emotional regulation mechanisms.

5. Conclusion

The adolescents with conduct disorder reported a low level of emotional distress and negative dysfunctional emotions (depression, anxiety) confirming the lack of a relationship between the symptoms of internalization and those of externalization with acts of aggression. Girls reported a higher level of emotional distress than boys, especially on negative dysfunctional emotion depression and significantly lower positive emotions. We found significant correlations between the emotional distress reported by the adolescents and their irrational cognitions, the relations intensities varying from medium to high. We found no significant relation between emotional distress and the emotional regulation strategies reappraisal and suppression measured by ERQ. The use of suppression coping strategy related significantly with all domains measured by ICU (callousness, uncaring, and unemotional), the intensity varying from medium to high. The use of reappraisal coping strategy related significantly only with ICU uncaring and ICU total score, the relations being negative. Callousness traits related significantly with the irrationality subscale need for comfort and the uncaring traits with the self-downing irrationality subscale.

The multitude of information and approaches in conduct disorder research underline the need for a comprehensive and individualized approach to treatment, recognizing the different needs and vulnerabilities. It is important to correlate research findings from different areas with pathology in order to improve current therapies (i.e., including emotion regulation training individualized in intervention protocol) or developing new ones.

Conflict of interests

The authors declare that they have no conflict of interest.

Author details

Roxana Șipoș* and Elena Predescu

*Address all correspondence to: roxana.sipos@umfcluj.ro

"Iuliu Hatieganu" University of Medicine and Pharmacy Cluj-Napoca, Department of Neuroscience, Discipline of Psychiatry and Pediatric Psychiatry, Cluj-Napoca, Romania

References

[1] Polanczyk GV, Salum GA, Sugaya LS, Caye A, Rohde LA. Annual research review: A meta-analysis of the worldwide prevalence of mental disorders in children and adolescents. Journal of Child Psychology and Psychiatry. 2015;**56**(3):345-365. DOI: 10.1111/jcpp.12381

[2] Canino G, Polanczyk G, Bauermeister JJ, Rohde LA, Frick PJ. Does the prevalence of CD and ODD vary across cultures? Social Psychiatry and Psychiatric Epidemiology. 2010;**45**(7):695-704. DOI: 10.1007/s00127-010-0242-y

[3] Romeo R, Knapp M, Scott S. Economic cost of severe antisocial behaviour in children – and who pays it. British Journal of Psychiatry. 2006;**188**:547-553

[4] Olesen J, Gustavsson A, Svensson M, Wittchen HU, Jönsson B. CDBE2010 study group; European brain council. The economic cost of brain disorders in Europe. European Journal of Neurology. 2012;**19**(1):155-162. DOI: 10.1111/j.1468-1331.2011.03590.x

[5] Lahey BB, Loeber R, Hart EL, Frick PJ, Applegate B, Zhang Q, Green SM, Russo MF. Four-year longitudinal study of conduct disorder in boys: Patterns and predictors of persistence. Journal of Abnormal Child Psychology. 1995;**104**(1):83-93

[6] American Psychiatric Association, editor. Diagnostic and Statistical Manual of Mental Disorders. 5th ed. Washington, DC: Author; 2013

[7] World Health Organization, editor. The ICD-10 Classification of Mental and Behavioural Disorders: Clinical Descriptions and Diagnostic Guidelines. Geneva: World Health Organization; 1992

[8] Moffitt TE. Adolescence-limited and life-course-persistent antisocial behavior: A developmental taxonomy. Psychological Review. 1993;**100**(4):674-701

[9] Moffitt TE. Life-course persistent versus adolescence-limited antisocial behaviour. In: Cicchetti D, Cohen J, editors. Developmental Psychopathology, 2nd Edition: Risk, Disorder, and Adaptation. 2nd ed. New York: Wiley; 2006. p. 570-598

[10] Frick PJ, Dickens C. Current perspectives on conduct disorder. Current Psychiatry Reports. 2006;**8**(1):59-72

[11] Kahn RE, Frick PJ, Youngstrom E, Findling RL, Youngstrom JK. The effects of including a callous unemotional specifier for the diagnosis of conduct disorder. Journal of Child Psychology and Psychiatry, and Allied Disciplines. 2012;**53**(3):271-282. DOI: 10.1111/j.1469-7610.2011.02463.x.

[12] Rowe R, Maughan B, Moran P, Ford T, Briskman J, Goodman R. The role of callous and unemotional traits in the diagnosisof conduct disorder. Journal of Child Psychology and Psychiatry. 2010;**51**(6):688-695

[13] Herpers PC, Rommelse NN, Bons DM, Buitelaar JK, Scheepers FE. Callous-unemotional traits as a cross-disorders con-struct. Social Psychiatry and Psychiatric Epidemiology. 2012;**9**:1-20

[14] Frick PJ, Marsee MA. Psychopaty and developmental pathways to antisocial behaviour in youth. In: Patrick CJ, editor. The Handbook of Psychopathy. New York: Guilford Press; 2006. p. 353-375

[15] Lahey BB, Waldman ID. Annual research review: Phe-notypic and causal structure of conduct disorder in the broadercontext of prevalent forms of psychopathology. Journal of Child Psychology and Psychiatry. 2012;**53**(5):536-557

[16] Frick PJ, Stickle TR, Dandreaux DM, Farrell JM, Kimonis ER. Callous-unemotional traits in predicting the severity and stability of conduct problems and delinquency. Journal of Abnormal Child Psychology. 2005;**33**:471-487

[17] Burke JD, Loeber R, Lahey BB. Adolescent conduct disorder and interpersonal callousness as predictors of psychopathy in young adults. Journal of Clinical Child & Adolescent Psychology. 2007;**36**(3):334-346

[18] Fergusson DM, Horwood LJ, Ridder EM. Show me the child at seven: The consequences of conduct problems in childhood for psychosocial functioning in adulthood. Journal of Child Psychology and Psychiatry. 2005;**46**(8):837-849

[19] Eisenbarth H, Demetriou C, Kyranides MN, Fanti K. Stability subtypes of callous–unemotional traits and conduct disorder symptoms and their correlates. Journal of Youth and Adolescence. 2016;**45**(9):1889-1901. DOI: 10.1007/s10964-016-0520-4

[20] Fanti KA, Panayiotou G, Lombardo MV, Kyranides MN. Unemotional on all counts: Evidence of reduced affective responses in individuals with high callous-unemotional traits across emotion systems and valences. Social Neuroscience. 2016;**11**(1):72-87. DOI: 10.1080/17470919.2015.1034378

[21] Fanti KA. Individual, social, and behavioral factors associated with co-occurring conduct problems and callous-unemotional traits. Journal of Abnormal Child Psychology. 2013;**41**(5):811-824. DOI: 10.1007/s10802-013-9726-z

[22] Kahn RE, Frick PJ, Youngstrom EA, Youngstrom JK, Feeny NC, Findling RL. Distinguishing primary and secondary variants of callous unemotional traits among adolescents in a clinic-referred sample. Psychological Assessment. 2013;**25**(3):966-978. DOI: 10.1037/a0032880

[23] Loney BR, Frick PJ, Clements CB, Ellis ML, Kerlin K. Callous-unemotional traits, impulsivity, and emotional processing in adolescents with antisocial behavior problems. Journal of Clinical Child and Adolescent Psychology. 2003;**32**(1):66-80

[24] Lemerise EA, Arsenio WF. An integrated model of emotion processes and cognition in social information processing. Child Development. 2000;**71**(1):107-118

[25] Hubbard JA, Smithmyer CM, Ramsden SR, Parker EH, Flanagan KD, Dearing KF, et al. Observational, physiological, and self-report measures of children's anger: Relations to reactive versus proactive aggression. Child Development. 2002;**73**:1101-1118

[26] Kimonis ER, Frick PJ, Fazekas H, Loney BR. Psychopathy, aggression, and the processing of emotional stimuli in non-referred girls and boys. Behavioral Sciences & The Law. 2006;**24**(1):21-37

[27] Muñoz LC, Frick PJ, Kimonis ER, Aucoin KJ. Types of aggression, responsiveness to provocation, and callous-unemotional traits in detained adolescents. Journal of Abnormal Child Psychology. 2008;**36**(1):15-28

[28] Sharp C, Vanwoerden S, Van Baardewijk Y, Tackett JL, Stegge H. Callous-unemotional traits are associated with deficits in recognizing complex emotions in preadolescent children. Journal of Personality Disorders. 2015;**29**(3):347-359

[29] Smith CA, Lazarus RS. Appraisal components, core relational themes, and the emotions. Cognition and Emotion. 1993;**7**:233-269

[30] Gross JJ, John OP. Individual differences in two emotion regulation processes: Implications for affect, relationships, and well-being. Journal of Personality and Social Psychology. 2003;**85**(2):348-362

[31] Sullivan TN, Helms SW, Kliewer W, Goodman KL. Associations between sadness and anger regulatin coping, emotional expression, and psysical and relational aggression among urban adolescents. Social Development. 2010;**19**(1):30-51

[32] Norström T, Pape H. Innovative but insufficient? A response to graham's commentary on 'alcohol, suppressed anger and violence. Addiction. 2010;**105**(12):2219-2220. DOI: 10.1111/j.1360-0443.2010.03221.x

[33] Roberton T, Daffern M, Bucks R. Emotion regulation and aggression. Aggresion and Violent Behavior. 2012;**17**:72-82

[34] Tull MT, Jakupcak M, Paulson A, Gratz KL. The role of emotional inexpressivity and experiential avoidance in the relationship between posttraumatic stress disorder symptom severity and aggressive behavior among men exposed to interpersonal violence. Anxiety, Stress, and Coping. 2007;**20**(4):337-351

[35] Szasz PL, Szentagotai A, Hofmann SG. The effect of emotion regulation strategies on anger. Behaviour Research and Therapy. 2010;**49**(2):114-119

[36] Pardini D, Frick PJ. Multiple developmental pathways to conduct disorder: Current conceptualizations and clinical implications. Journal of the Canadian Academy of Child and Adolescent Psychiatry. 2013;**22**(1):20-25

[37] National Institute for Health and Care Excellence, NICE. Antisocial behaviour and conduct disorders in children and young people: recognition and management [Internet]. 2013. Available from: http://www nice org uk/guidance/cg158 [Last accessed 30 November 2015]. [Accessed: 12 August 2017]

[38] Ellis A. Reason and Emotion in Psychotherapy, Revised and Updated. Secaucus, NJ: Carol Publishing Group; 1994

[39] David D, Szentagotai A. Cognitions in cognitive-behavioral psychotherapies; toward an integrative model. Clinical Psychology Review. 2006;**26**:284-298

[40] Fives CJ, Kong G, Fuller JR, DiGiuseppe R. Anger, aggression, and irrational beliefs in adolescents. Cognitive Therapy and Research. 2011;**35**:199-208

[41] Hawes DJ, Dadds MR. The treatment of conduct problems in children with callous-unemotional traits. Journal of Consulting and Clinical Psychology. 2005;**73**(4):737-741

[42] Hipwell A, Keenan K, Kasza K, Loeber R, Stouthamer-Loeber M, Bean T. Reciprocal influences between girls' conduct problems and depression, and parental punishment and warmth: A six year prospective analysis. Journal of Abnormal Child Psychology. 2008;**36**(5):663-677

[43] Pardini DA, Lochman JE, Frick PJ. Callous/unemotional traits and social-cognitive processes in adjudicated youths. Journal of the American Academy of Child and Adolescent Psychiatry. 2003;**42**(3):364-371

[44] Layard R, Clark DM, editors. Thrive: The Power of Evidence-based Psychological Therapies. London: Allen Lane; 2014

[45] Buitelaar JK, Smeets KC, Herpers P, Scheepers F, Glennon J, Rommelse NN. Conduct disorders. European Child & Adolescent Psychiatry. 2013;**22**(1):S49-S54. DOI: 10.1007/s00787-012-0361-y

[46] Opris D, Macavei B. The profile of emotional distress; norms for the romanian population. Journal of Cognitive and Behavioral Psychotherapies. 2007;**7**:139-157

[47] Lindner H, Kirkby R, Wertheim E, Birch PA. Brief assessment of irrational thinking: The shortened general attitude and belief scale. Cognitive Therapy and Research. 1999;**23**(6):651-663

[48] Trip S. Scala de atitudini şi convingeri generale, forma scurta – GABS-SV (trad.). In: David D, editor. Sistem de evaluare clinică. Cluj-Napoca: RTS; 2007

[49] Macavei B, McMahon J. The assessment of rational and irrational beliefs. In: David D, Lynn SJ, Ellis A, editors Rational and Irrational Beliefs: Research, Theory, and Clinical Practice. New York, NY: Oxford. pp. 115-147

[50] Sava FA, Maricuţoiu LP, Rusu S, Vîrgă D, Macsinga I. Implicit and explicit self esteem and irrational beliefs. Journal of Cognitive and Behavioral Psychotherapies. 2011;**11**(1):97-111

[51] Ellis A. Rational Emotive Behavior Therapy: It Works for me; it can Work for you. Amherst, NY: Prometheus Books; 2004

[52] Vernon A. Rational Emotive Behavior Therapy over Time. Washington, DC: American Psychological Association; 2010

[53] Ellis A, Ellis DJ. Rational Emotive Behavior Therapy. Washington, DC: American Psychological Association; 2011

[54] Frick PJ, Cornell AH, Barry CT, Bodin SD, Dane HE. Callous-unemotional traits and conduct problems in the prediction of conduct problem severity, aggression, and self-report of delinquency. Journal of Abnormal Child Psychology. 2003;**31**:457-470

[55] Frick PJ, Bodin SD, Barry CT. Psychopathic traits and conduct problems in community and clinic-referred samples of children: Further development of the psychopathy screening device. Psychological Assessment. 2000;**12**:382-393

[56] Katz LF, Windecker-Nelson B. Parental meta-emotion philosophy in families with conduct-problem children: Links with peer relationships. Journal of Abnormal Child Psychology. 2004;**32**:385-398. DOI: 10.1023/B:JACP.0000030292.36168.30

[57] Fainsilber Katz L, Windecker-Nelson B. Parental meta-emotion philosophy in families with conduct-problem children: Links with peer relations. Journal of Abnormal Child Psychology. 2004;**32**(4):385-398

[58] Calkins SD, Dedmon SE. Physiological and behavioral regulation in two-year-old children with aggressive/destructive behavior problems. Journal of Abnormal Child Psychology. 2000;**28**:103-118

[59] Calvete E, Cardeñoso O. Gender differences in cognitive vulnerability to depression and behavior problems in adolescents. Journal of Abnormal Child Psychology. 2005; **33**:179-192

[60] Gross JJ, Levenson RW. Emotional suppression – physiology, self-report, and expressive behavior. Journal of Personality and Social Psychology. 1993;**64**(6):970-986

[61] Hofmann SG, Asmundson GJG. Acceptance and mindfulness-based therapy: New wave or old hat? Clinical Psychology Review. 2008;**28**(1):1-16

[62] Hayes SC, Strosahl KD, Wilson KG. Acceptance and Commitment Therapy: An Experiential Approach to Behavior Change. New York: Guilford Press; 1999

[63] Linehan M. Cognitive Behavioral Treatment for Borderline Personality Disorder. New York: Guilford Press; 1993

[64] Segal ZV, Williams JMG, Teasdale JD. Mindfulness-based Cognitive Therapy for Depression: A New Approach to Preventing Relapse. New York: Guilford Press; 2002

[65] Steinberg L, Blatt-Eisengart I, Cauffman E. Patterns of competence and adjustment among adolescents from authoritative, authoritarian, indulgent, and neglectful homes: A replication in a sample of serious juvenile offenders. Journal of Research on Adolescence. 2006;**16**:47-58. DOI: 10.1111/j.1532-7795.2006.00119.x

[66] Eisenberg N, Hofer C, Vaughan J. Effortful control and its socioemotional consequences. In: Gross JJ, editor. Handbook of Emotion Regulation. New York: The Guilford Press; 2007. p. 229-248

[67] Eisenberg N, Spinrad TL, Eggum ND, Silva KM, Reiser M, Hofer C, Michalik N. Relations among maternal socialization, effortful control, and maladjustment in early childhood. Development and Psychopathology. 2010;**22**:507-525. DOI: 10.1017/S0954579410000246

[68] Blair RJJ. The neurobiology of psychopathic traits in youths. Nature Reviews Neuroscience. 2013;**14**(11):786-799. DOI: 10.1038/nrn3577

[69] Frick PJ. Unpublished rating scale. University of New Orleans; 2004. Inventory of callous-unemotional traits.

[70] Moretti MM, Holland R, McKay S. Self-other representations and relational and overt aggression in adolescent girls and boys. Behavioral Sciences & The Law. 2001;**19**:109-126

[71] Spinrad TL, Eisenberg N, Cumberland A, Fabes RA, Valiente C, Shepard SA, Reiser M, Losoya SH, Guthrie IK. Relation of emotion-related regulation to children's social competence: A longitudinal study. Emotion. 2006;**6**(3):498-510

Chapter 5

Cognitive-Behavioral Theory and Treatment of Antisocial Personality Disorder

Ahmet Emre Sargın, Kadir Özdel and
Mehmet Hakan Türkçapar

Additional information is available at the end of the chapter

http://dx.doi.org/10.5772/intechopen.68986

Abstract

Antisocial personality disorder (ASPD) has a distinct cognitive profile according to cognitive theory of personality disorders. Antisocial individuals' view of the world is personal rather than interpersonal. They cannot accept another's point of view over their own. As such, they cannot take on the role of another. Their actions are not based on choices in a social sense because of this cognitive limitation. Cognitive theory of personality disorders conceptualizes personality disorder including the ASPD, according to their basic beliefs or schemas. The content of beliefs can vary in different personality disorders. Antisocial patients view themselves as loners, autonomous, and strong. Some of them see themselves as having been abused and mistreated by society and therefore justify victimizing others because they believe that they have been victimized. Their view about other people is very negative; they see others as exploitative and thus deserving of being exploited in retaliation. In this chapter, after overviewing general features of ASPD, we aim to give an explanation how cognitive behavioral therapy (CBT) conceptualizes personality disorders in general and ASPD in particular and highlight the important implementations of CBT and schema therapy.

Keywords: antisocial personality disorder, cognitive behavioral theory

1. Introduction

Antisocial personality disorder (ASPD) is defined as a pervasive pattern of disregard and violation of the right of others [1]. Patients with ASPD often have problems with judiciary system like being arrested or imprisoned because they do not respect the right of others, they have tendency to violate the laws, anger problems, and alcohol/substance addiction [2].

During psychiatric interview they may seem inoffensive and even little bit charming but under this mask of sanity there is aggression, hostility, rage, and tension. They have defensiveness when replying the self-report scales [3]. During their lifetime, they repeatedly exhibit traits of impulsivity, low conscientiousness, which cause social and interpersonal problems. They may repeatedly perform illegal acts, lie or malinger people. They are manipulative in order to gain personal profit or pleasure. They disregard the feelings or wishes of others. Due to their impulsivity, they may change their jobs, accommodation or relationships all of a sudden without taking into consideration of the consequences. They are irresponsible as a partner and as a parent. They frequently have more than one sexual partner and hardly sustain monogamous relationships. Their children generally live in bad conditions such as lack of hygiene, malnutrition, or accommodation. All these disadvantages result in high rates of unemployment, bad housing, and being imprisoned and dying prematurely due to reckless behavior [4, 5].

The two main diagnostic systems, Diagnostic and Statistical Manual of Mental Disorders (DSM-5) and WHO's International Statistical Classification of Diseases and Related Health Problems, 10th edition (ICD-10), have similar criteria for antisocial personality construct.

According to the latest version of Diagnostic and Statistical Manual of Mental Disorders (DSM-5), ASPD is conceptualized through a criterion set which includes criminal behavior, lying, reckless and impulsive behavior, aggression and irresponsibility [4]. Although it defines a similar construct, the diagnostic label for antisocial personality has different name in ICD-10, as dissocial personality disorder. Dissocial personality disorder is defined in ICD-10 as characterized by disregard for social obligations, and callous unconcern for the feelings of others. There is gross disparity between behavior and the prevailing social norms. Behavior is not readily modifiable by adverse experience, including punishment. There is a low tolerance for frustrationand and a low threshold for discharge of aggression, including violence; there is a tendency to blame others or to offer plausible rationalizations for the behavior bringing the patient into conflict with society.

The two classifications are not identical but similar. The ICD-10 emphasizes the impairment in the interpersonal and the affective domain while DSM-5 focuses merely on the antisocial behaviour. (For instance there is a criteria of low tolerance for frustration, low threshold for aggression and violence in ICD-10 whereas DSM-5 focuses merely impulsivity, disregard for others, and irresponsible behaviors.) Also conduct disorder before the age of 15 is not necessary in ICD-10 criteria.

Antisocial personality like clinical entity is first defined as "moral insanity" in nineteenth century by Dr. J.C. Prichard in England. The moral insanity term is later replaced by another term psychopathy [6]. Psychopathy is first defined in "The mask of sanity" book of Cleckley and later conceptualized by Hare with the psychopathy checklist-revised (PCL-R) [7, 8]. Psychopathy is accepted as more severe than ASPD or dissocial personality disorder. It generally includes remorselessness, deceitfulness, egocentricity, superficial charm to others, depression and anxiety, and externalization of blame [9]. The psychopaths generally have lack of fear to aversive events and a deficit in processing affective information regardless of whether it is positive or negative [10]. There are studies suggesting that psychopaths have deficiency in empathy [11].

The prevalence of ASPD varies from depending on the instruments, methodology, and the country. It is between 1.3 and 6.8% for men and 0 and 0.8% for women [5, 12]. The prevalence is higher in populations that are affected by low socioeconomic factors. The ratio of men/women is 3. Approximately 50–80% of the criminals meet the diagnostic criteria of ASPD [13, 14]. Patients with ASPD may also have comorbid substance use disorders, anxiety disorders, depressive disorders, somatic symptoms and impulse control problems such as gambling disorder [5, 15, 16].

Like most of the psychiatric disorders, antisocial personality disorder is a heterogeneous diagnosis which has both biological and psychological etiology. From the adoption studies, it is seen that a child who has genetic vulnerability living in an adverse environment is prone to ASPD [17].

It was also asserted that psychopaths may have lack of cortical physiological responses that are associated with experiencing feelings, especially fear. Accordingly, some studies determined that psychopaths do not have autonomic hyperarousal when faced with a provoking stimulus unlike people without ASPD [18, 19].

On the other hand, according to cognitive behavioral theory it is assumed that there is developmental delay in the moral maturity and cognitive functioning of antisocial individuals which we will focus on the next chapter deeply [20].

2. Cognitive behavioral theory of antisocial personality disorder

2.1. Cognitive behavioral theory

When conceptualizing the human behaviour, cognitions and emotions, cognitive model views the cognition under two main titles: Automatic thoughts and schemas. Automatic thoughts are cognitions that accompany the distressful emotions and are specific to that situation/activating event. They are not the product of directed/driven thoughts that are created after a willing process. They rather pop up suddenly and the individuals mostly do not notice the automatic thought but the emotion resulting from it. They do not follow grammatical rules but rather they are set of meanings or images (i.e., "I am a bad mother," or having an image of himself/herself lying in bed in emergency service) flowing in the mind which are immediately accepted without evaluation by the individual and cause a distressful emotion [21, 22]. So when an activating event (A) occurs, this leads to a cognition, interpretation, evaluation, an automatic thought which is merely maladaptive/functional (B) and this leads to an emotion and a behaviour (C). Accordingly, the cognitive behavioral model emphasizes that it is not the event/situation that determines how the individual feels or behaves (**Figure 1**). It is the interpretation of that event/situation that determines the feelings and behaviors. This is why cognitive behavioral therapists suggest disputing these maladaptive/dysfunctional thoughts to modify emotions [23].

Schemas are divided into two domains: core beliefs and intermediate beliefs (underlying rules and assumptions). Although some authors like Padesky have used the term schema only to describe core beliefs; in general, core beliefs are included as a domain of schema along

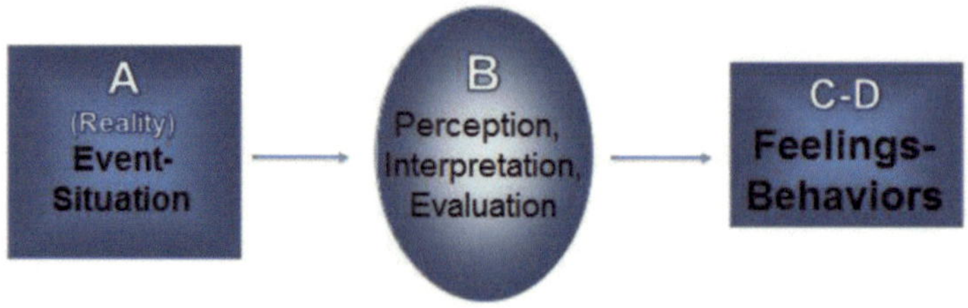

Figure 1. ABC model of cognitive behavioral therapy.

with intermediate beliefs [24]. Core beliefs are the cognitive constructs that determine how to regulate the information about himself/herself and his/her environment and include the essential assumptions about himself/herself, the others, and the world. After being developed as a result of early life experiences/memories and identifications with the important figures, core beliefs are reinforced with the similar experiences and learnings throughout the years [22, 25]. These beliefs about self and life constitute the emotional and behavioral traits of personality. These beliefs are so rigid, fundamental, and deep that even the individual himself/herself does not articulate them. The individual accepts these ideas as undisputable truths. Beck divides the core beliefs in three [25]:

(1) Unlovable core beliefs: "I am unlovable," "I am unattractive," "I am rejected," "I am not desired," "I am ugly," etc.

(2) Helpless core beliefs: "I am weak," "I am incompetent," "I am passive," "I am a loser," "I am coward," etc.

(3) Worthless core beliefs: "I am worthless," "I am bad," "I am disgusting," "I deserve to be punished," "I am guilty," etc.

Core beliefs exist in pairs in all the humans. For example, an individual has both "I am lovable" and "I am not lovable" core beliefs. A healthy person who does not have a psychiatric disorder or a personality disorder has the positive core belief as the effective trait ("I am lovable"). When the healthy individual experiences a negative event, the negative core belief gets activated. For example, when a healthy person breaks up from his/her partner, the core belief "I am not lovable" gets activated. This person may feel down for a while or he/she may have depression for a period. But when he/she gets rid of depression, the positive core belief becomes active. If the individual has chronic depression or a personality disorder, this means that the positive core belief is very weak. It is generally the negative core belief dominant in his/her life. As a result he/she is not able to get rid of what that core belief ("I am not lovable") is imposing. This kind of person only accepts the data confirming the negative core belief and discounts the data that does not fit into the schema. The negative core belief is like a broadcasting radio that never stops telling how much unlovable he/she is.

Underneath the superficial automatic thoughts, there lie the intermediate beliefs, rules, and assumptions. These rules, beliefs, and assumptions are the abstract regulators of the behaviour although they are not verbalized by the individual. They are settled rules, expectations, and attitudes about the individual himself/herself, the others or the world/experiences (i.e., "If I cry, it means that I am a weak person," "I must do everything perfect so that people would not understand I am actually incompetent"). Intermediate beliefs are the interconnections between the core beliefs and the automatic thoughts. Their functions are:

- Maintaining the core belief by bringing an explanation to the life experiences which are in contradiction with the core beliefs. For instance, an individual has a belief of "All human beings are bad." When this person comes across with someone who treats him/her in a good manner, he runs into a contradiction with his/her core belief. In order to overcome this contradiction, the individual comes up with the intermediate belief "If someone treats me well that means that he/she has an axe to grind."
- Having a life compatible with the core belief: If a person has a core belief of incompetency, he/she avoids taking any risks.
- Protecting the individual from the intense affect that arises from the activation of the core belief. For instance, if a person has a core belief of worthlessness, in order not to confront this core belief, the individual grabs to the intermediate belief: "If I become successful at work, I will be worthful."

Intermediate beliefs can be determined by determining the common and repeating themes in the automatic thoughts, by asking the meaning and the possible consequences of the automatic thought (downward arrow technique), or patient filling some scales (i.e., dysfunctional attitudes scale—DAS) [22].

To sum up, cognitive behavioral model assumes that we all have core beliefs that are rooted from genetic disposition and early childhood experiences. These core beliefs determine our intermediate beliefs (assumptions, rules, attitudes). Together these two are called schema. Schemas are kind of reservoir, which has explanations, assumptions, and strategies about the individual, others, and the world. When an activating event occurs, automatic thoughts are generated from this reservoir and shape feelings and behaviors (**Figure 2**). What cognitive

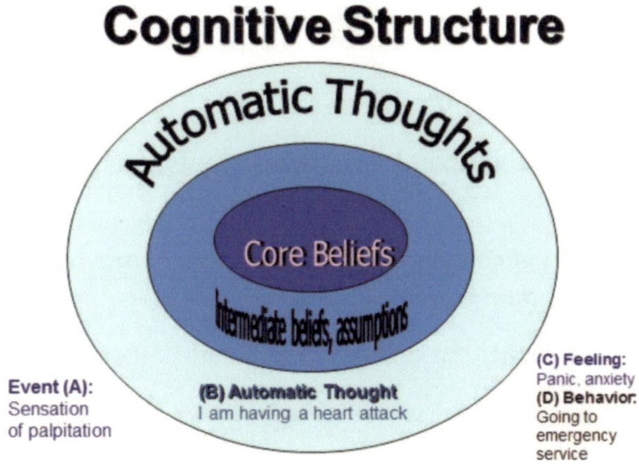

Figure 2. Cognitive structure.

behavioral therapy does, is to decrease the distressful emotions by disputing the maladaptive dysfunctional automatic thoughts first, and drying the reservoir (schemas) which from which these thoughts generate in the long run if the client frequently/chronically gets effected by these schemas. In cognitive behavioral therapy, cognitive processes can be integrated with the behavioral strategies to optimize the learning process.

Let us consider a person who has antisocial personality disorder and when this person gets across with new people he/she may have thoughts of cheating or giving harm. These thoughts may come from the intermediate beliefs of "I must be the one who hits first, otherwise I will be the loser," "Other people are nothing but wimps and they exist in life for being cheated/deceived," or "Laws are impediments for a satisfactory life and they are for weak people, if I obey the laws I will be exploited by other people." Of course these beliefs may be very well reflection of the core belief "I am weak and I may get hurt."

Today, with many schools focusing on the different components (i.e., schema therapy, dialectical behavioral therapy, acceptance, and commitment therapy, mindfulness based cognitive therapy) cognitive behavioral therapy (CBT)is found to be effective in numerous psychiatric disorders/psychological problems like depression, obsessive-compulsive disorder, panic disorder, generalized anxiety disorder, personality disorders, eating disorders, couple problems, family problems, and anger control problems [26–30].

2.2. Schema concept according to Young

Similar to cognitive behavioral therapy, Jeffrey Young stated that schemas develop in childhood in response to genetic predisposition and some environmental influences. Young viewed schema as resulting from unmet emotional needs in childhood [31]. To explain these unhelpful schemas, he introduced the concept of early maladaptive schemas (EMSs). According to Young, EMSs are unconditional and dysfunctional beliefs about the self. Like the adaptive schemas, EMSs develop from early experiences with the parents, caretakers, or peers during the childhood. A child who is not able to get his/her basic needs actualized; he/she develops schemas as the coping mechanisms to make sense of the experience and the world around him/her [32]. Young has delineated 18 schemas in five domains. These domains reflect the basic emotional needs of the child. The domains and the early maladaptive schemas are listed below [31]:

(a) **Disconnection and rejection:** Abandonment/instability, mistrust/abuse, emotional deprivation, defectiveness/shame, social isolation/alienation

(b) **Impaired autonomy and performance:** Dependence/incompetence, vulnerability to harm or illness, enmeshment/undeveloped self, failure

(c) **Impaired limits:** Entitlement/grandiosity, insufficient self-control/self-discipline

(d) **Other-directedness:** Subjugation, self-sacrifice, approval-seeking/recognition-seeking

(e) **Overvigilance and inhibition:** Negativity/pessimism, emotional inhibition, unrelenting standards/hypercriticalness, punitiveness

Because each schema has interpersonal, cognitive, and affective components, and it gives a perspective to the individual about the unmet needs that are experienced during early childhood; when EMSs are activated, high levels of affects show up causing significant distress and even psychiatric disorders. To overcome this distress, the individual may choose three options. Whichever option he/she chooses, he/she may decrease the intense affect, but the schema will be reinforced anyway. According to Young, these three options are [31]:

(1) **Schema maintenance:** Individuals, who have schema maintenance, accept the schema as completely true. Although they experience the negative emotions provoked by the schema, they keep on behaving in a way to confirm the schema. In their adulthood, they re-experience the similar traumas which created that schema. This type of behaviour is like taking the same action and hoping for a different outcome desperately.

(2) **Schema avoidance:** In this type of maladaptive coping mechanism, the individual completely tries to ignore the schema. They try not to think or feel anything that has a potential to trigger schema. In order to avoid the schema, they may spend their time to distract themselves like alcohol, etc. Similarly, they have a tendency to avoid therapy and to face these disturbing thoughts and feelings about their schema. It is not uncommon for these kinds of clients to engage in therapy interfering behaviors like being late or not doing the homework. This type of behaviour is like burying one's head in the sand like an ostrich.

(3) **Schema compensation**: Schema compensation means behaving in a way that the schema does not exist at all. At first glance, it may seem like a healthy mechanism but what the client does is merely an overcompensation effort to camouflage the schema beneath. This overcompensation effort may likely cause affective and interpersonal problems. Metaphorically speaking, this coping mechanism resembles a balloon being overinflated and blowing out ultimately. An example could be a person who has a schema of mistrust/abuse abusing others.

Having defined these concepts, Young developed schema therapy which has some adaptations cognitive behavioral therapy, psychodynamic therapy, and gestalt therapy. Because an individual always has more than one schema and there is always a shift from one schema to another in response to activating event, Young defined modes. A mode is a state of mind consisting of many schemas, coping behaviors in reaction to these schemas and the emotions. A mode can be maladaptive or healthy. An individual has many different modes and with result of the activating event, one of these modes get activated while others remain silent. As a new activating event occurs, another mode becomes active. To sum up, at any given time there is an active mode in an individual and due to the activating events there is always a shift from one mode to another.

Young defined the modes under four headings: child modes, coping modes, parent modes, and the healthy adult mode [31].

Child modes: There are four child modes. These are vulnerable child, angry child, impulsive/undisciplined child, and the contented child. Vulnerable child is characterized by the emotions of sadness, anguish, and shame. It includes subtypes of "lonely child," "abandoned and abused child," and "humiliated and inferior child" while angry child mode has subtypes of "stubborn child" and "enraged child". The last one "contended child" is the mode in which the basic needs of the child are met. Child modes are assumed to be universal and congenital [33].

Maladaptive coping modes: These modes are compliant surrenderer, detached protector, and overcompensator.

Parent modes: Because schemas come into existence because of the basic needs not implemented, or aversive experiences such as trauma, neglect, or abuse, parental modes usually derive from attachment figures which can be parents or anyone else (peers, social authority, etc.). While overwhelming emotions dominate the child modes, clients experience parental modes as negative thoughts. There are two parent modes: punitive parent and demanding parent.

Healthy adult: This is the aim of the schema therapy to accomplish ultimately. A healthy adult is able to set limits and/or accept and embrace the unhealthy maladaptive modes besides function in domains of social/family and occupational life.

The strategy in schema therapy is once modes are identified, the therapist and the client challenge the current maladaptive modes to deactivate it. After the deactivation, more adaptive and functional mode is introduced with some cognitive and experiential techniques which we will mention in the following chapters [33]. During this process, after identifying early maladaptive schemas, it is crucial to notice and validate the client's unmet emotional needs. Changing early maladaptive schemas to more adaptive and functional, adaptive schemas must be necessarily accompanied by changing maladaptive coping skills and replacing them with more appropriate ones.

Schema therapy has been investigated in many personality disorders but most of the studies were conducted about the efficacy in borderline personality disorder. Studies found that schema therapy was superior to treatment as usual and some other psychotherapy approaches with lower dropout rate and more cost effective [34–36]. In a study conducted by Bamelis et al., schema therapy was compared with clarification oriented psychotherapy (COP) and treatment as usual group in terms of clinical effectiveness and economical cost effectiveness-cost utility in six personality disorders (avoidant, dependent, obsessive-compulsive, paranoid, histrionic, and narcissistic). The study was conducted in 12 mental health institutes with 323 patients. It was found that schema therapy was more effective and had less dropout rates compared to treatment as usual or COP [37].

2.3. Cognitive behavioral theory of antisocial personality disorder

Although Young schema questionnaire (YSQ) scores are generally found to be higher in clients with personality disorders, there is still insufficient evidence to identify specific schemas for specific disorders. In the study that was conducted by Jovev and Jackson, it was aimed to examine which of the schema domains are specific in three personality disorders. For borderline personality disorder, high scores on dependence/incompetence, defectiveness/shame, and abandonment schema domains were detected while elevations on unrelenting standards and emotional inhibition schema domains were associated with obsessive-compulsive personality disorder and avoidant personality disorder, respectively [38]. While Nordahl et al. found that vulnerability to harm, emotional inhibition, and insufficient self-control were associated with narcissistic personality disorder [39], in their nonclinical sample, Reeves and Taylor found that men endorsed more symptoms of ASPD and higher levels of the core beliefs of emotional deprivation, social isolation, defectiveness/shame, and emotional inhibition [40].

The traditional view of ASPD is that these people have deficiency in internalizing the standards of the society [41]. Beck and Freeman suggest that there is evidence for developmental delay in moral maturity and cognitive functioning of antisocial individuals [20]. They have poor empathic ability and they are not able to perceive other people's point of view. They see themselves as loners, autonomous, and strong, and some of them may see themselves as abused and mistreated by society. They see others as either exploitative or weak and vulnerable [25].

According to Millon and Everly, antisocial individuals tend to be interpersonally aggressive, abusive, and cruel. They have learned to rely on themselves and to distrust others because they have a fear of being exploited and humiliated by others. They are secured only when they are in control of the situation and are independent of the will of others who may threaten their security (e.g., interpersonal control) [42].

When we look at the relation between the EMS and the aggressive behaviour, we see that Tremblay and Dozois found a relation between the domain of disconnection and rejection (abandonment, mistrust/abuse, social isolation) and domain of impaired limits (entitlement, insufficient self-control) and trait aggressiveness [43]. Gilbert and colleagues aimed to find out the prevalence of EMSs in offenders and they determined that entitlement, social isolation, dependence, insufficient self-control, and failure to achieve are associated with aggression [44]. Loper et al. investigated the relation between the schemas and the personality disorders in 116 incarcerated women who were convicted from robbery to assault. According to results, impaired limits presented with a sense of entitlement, poor impulse control, and lack of concern for others were correlated with cluster-B personality disorders including antisocial personality. This domain was also associated with hostility, institutional misconduct, self-reported violence, and victimization [45].

Polaschek and colleagues analyzed the interviews of the violent offenders and they identified implicit theories—a term which they define as structured interconnected belief network that guides behaviour and allows the individual to predict the result of a particular event [46]—instead of schema. From the transcript of the interview of the offenders, they uncovered four implicit theories: (1) beat or beaten, (2) I am the law, (3) violence is normal, and (4) I get out of control which corresponds to entitlement, mistrust/abuse, and insufficient self-control [47].

Ozdel et al. examined 38 patients diagnosed antisocial personality disorder selected from young soldiers most of whom were having substance abuse treatment in the army and 24 nonclinical volunteers. The purpose of the study was to identify core beliefs and early maladaptive schemas that characterize antisocial personality disorder. Diagnosis was made according to structured clinical interview for DSM-III-R personality disorders (SCID-II), Young schema questionnaire (YSQ), and the social comparison scale (SCS). SCS tries to identify judgments concerned with rank (inferior-superior) and determines how a person judges himself/herself as fitting in with or being similar to others. When the SCS scores of two groups were compared, it was found that there was a significant difference favoring the control group on these items: unlovable-lovable, lonely-not lonely, rejected-accepted, etc. In other words, control group subjects scored higher, meaning more positive social comparison perception. When the two groups were compared for YSQ, instead of simply comparing the means for specific schemas, the authors preferred to focus on schemas that showed significant differences and also had raw schema scores of 20 or more points. Using this procedure, significant findings were obtained for the specific schemas for emotional deprivation, entitlement/grandiosity, mistrust/abuse, vulnerability to harm, and social isolation. Three out of above five schemas-emotional deprivation, mistrust/abuse and social isolation fall into disconnection/rejection domain. Since this domain is conceptualized as stemming from a person's unmet needs for love, security, stability, and nurturance, it can be assumed that the current individual diagnosed with ASPD see himself/herself as unlovable, lonelier, and more rejected than the normal controls [48]. The results of SCS (the persons with ASPD tend to see themselves unlovable-lonely and rejected) supports the notion that antisocial persons may behave in order to compensate for a sense of victimization (ie., "I am weak so I must be the one who hits first."). Hence these findings may suggest that a conditional belief such as "I should hurt him before he hurts me" is behind the primary social strategies of attacking and exploiting used by individuals with ASPD [49]. This finding fits very well with the schema compensation strategy.

2.4. Treatment in antisocial personality disorder

When a therapist works with a client with antisocial personality disorder (ASPD) many challenges would be there from the beginning. First of all, most of the professionals believed that antisocial personality disorder is an untreatable condition. That's why they are reluctant to treat patients with ASPD. On the other side of the relationship antisocial patients that are coming for therapy are also very reluctant [50].

It is not common that an individual with ASPD goes to the therapist's office for getting help for the problems that are already considered so by the environment. They usually come to therapy when their conventional strategies have stopped working and have not been able to get what they wanted or the law or unofficial authority has threatened them. In these conditions, subjects of the admission are usually mood problems, behavioral problems, and alcohol and substance use problems. Another issue while working with ASPD is motivation. From the stages of change perspective, individuals with ASPD are usually at precontemplation or contemplation stages. This suggests that these people believe the source of the problem is from the outside; they are not the responsible one; or there is some kind of problem but they cannot do anything to solve it.

Above mentioned characteristics of the clinical picture of ASPD are also important guides to the therapist while working with them. This is all to say that the problem areas are mood problems including anger, anxiety, or depression; alcohol and substance use problems and the treatment strategy should consider teaching more functional attitudes and ways to get things wanted, and methods used in the treatment process must be motivational (i.e., pros and cons analysis).

Unfortunately, there is not any satisfactory evidence which therapeutic intervention is effective for antisocial personality disorder. In a meta-analysis searching for an effective therapy for ASPD concluded that although there are some interventions (i.e., contingency management with standard maintenance or CBT with standard maintenance, etc.) appeared to be effective for substance use problems, none of the psychological treatments were significantly effective [51].

Davidson et al. randomized 52 patients diagnosed with ASPD in two groups, one for CBT and one for treatment as usual. The CBT group received treatment either for 6 months or for 12 months. When the assessments made at baseline and at 12 months were compared, it was found that although 6 months of CBT decreased the problematic alcohol use and increased positive beliefs and social functioning more than the treatment as usual group, the difference was not significant [52].

From the cognitive behavioral point of view, treatment modalities are conventional CBT and schema therapy. Results of the studies used traditional CBT approaches are discouraging with nonsignificant behavioral changes and attitudes [53, 54]. However, a new cognitive behavioral model called the risk-need-responsivity (RNR) has become hope for the treatment of ASPD [55]. This approach assesses individuals with criminal and antisocial behavioral pattern based on their future risk of the criminal act, their needs, and environmental factors related to recidivism. In this approach, the aim is to reduce risk factors specifically connected lasting criminal behaviors since it is not usually used in untraditional mental health settings like prisons. The "risk" part of the model is about the intensity of the treatment because it is considered that the bigger the risk of future criminal behaviour, the more intense treatment is required. The "need" part of the model is about the goals of treatment. These goals are the ones that considered attempts of crimes mostly related to future. The "responsivity" part is about the consistency between the learning styles, ability, and motivational stages and interventions provided [56]. Since antisocial individuals have low motivation or learning abilities to change their somehow "working" strategies, completely individual treatment plan should be warranted. In this treatment plan, strategies pertaining to cognitive, behavioral, and social learning paradigms are used in order to construct an individual profile of learning. Andrew et al. proposed eight factors related to recidivism of the individuals with ASPD. In this risk-need-responsivity (RNR) model, risk factors are categorized under the two domains, which are static risk factors, such as previous crimes committed, and dynamic risk factors, such as current substance misuse. The main static risk factor is the history of antisocial behavior and the dynamic risk factors are disordered personality, criminal thinking (antisocial beliefs), antisocial associates, dysfunctional family or marital bonds, low levels of functioning and/or satisfaction in work/school, low levels of pro-social leisure activities, and substance abuse. Criminal thinking and disordered personality represent the focus for cognitive part of the therapeutic work. The other factors such as low family bond, unemployment, etc. represent the behavioral part of the therapy. Both cognitive and behavioral parts are sustained together. Antisocial personality beliefs can be assessed by an unstructured interview or some empirically supported tools such as personality belief questionnaire [57]. As for criminal thinking, there are various assessment tools for them. Once personality beliefs and criminal thinking aspects are found, cognitive interventions are implemented.

Cognitive interventions include introduction of conditional and unconditional beliefs; first cognitive restructuring of the intermediate beliefs in terms of rationality and functionality; positive schema log; and behavioral experiments.

Introduction of general CBT model and especially beliefs are of therapeutic effect. Attitudes, rules, and standards can be introduced as personal doctrines that can be hold or discharged according to their functionality and doctrine change would need time. Positive schema log is a cognitive technique in which client tries to detect concrete evidences contradicting to old core beliefs (these core beliefs can be about self or others). Behavioral experiments are well-designed individual experiments that try to test certain beliefs.

Behavioral interventions include functional analysis, self-monitoring, activity scheduling, and skills training (social skills training and assertiveness training).

Functional analysis is a work to examine triggers, behaviors, and the consequences of behaviors. These consequences are discussed in a short and long run. Intentions are not always in line with the consequences. This intervention has the individual focus on those consequences. Self-monitoring helps client to be able to stand back and observe him or herself. Activity scheduling helps clients to realize how they spend their times, which activities they usually engage in, and the effects of those activities. Skills training such as social skills training and assertiveness training should be better if added in treatment protocol when working with individuals with ASPD [58].

2.5. The basic concepts in schema therapy of antisocial personality disorder

As mentioned above, because antisocial personality disordered patients generally do not have enough motivation and referred to therapy for legal reasons, it is hard to keep them in therapy. Patients who have ASPD have very little concern about the consequences of their actions and how the others feel. They see themselves as lonely and victimized, so one of the most important things to move forward in therapy is to build a therapeutic rapport. Therapist uses two important strategies–limited reparenting and empathic confrontation–to build a relationship. ASPD patients have strong schemas due to their early childhood memories of unmet basic needs. Limited reparenting provides "corrective emotional experience" that feeds these unmet needs [59]. The responses, empathic attitude, and behaviors of the therapist construct the limited parenting in therapy sessions.

Empathic confrontation is another relational construct which is extremely useful during the change phase of the therapy. It is like a teeter–tooter. On one hand, the therapist accepts and shows the schema of the patient. He/she shows empathy about why the patient has that schema, what the utility of the schema was in the early childhood, and how it helped the patient to survive that traumatic period. On the other hand, the therapist confronts with the patient about the current consequences of the schema, how it destructs the patient's interpersonal relations, etc. Swinging between empathy and confrontation will lead the patient to be more open to alternative interpretations.

Cognitive strategies help the patient build a healthy adult mode, but before that the patient first has to realize his/her mode and then challenge it. It is very obvious that the patient will have difficulty in realizing his/her schema from many aspects; it is (was) a life-saving strategy for him/her. So cognitive strategies help the patient to step back and look at the picture from a distance. Cognitive strategies include [31]:

Testing the validity of a schema: It is like testing the validity of the automatic thoughts in CBT with the exception that, here the validity will be tested in considering the whole life rather than a particular situation. The therapist and the client search for the evidence for and against the schema.

Reframing the evidence supporting the schema: The therapist and the patient make a list of evidences supporting the schema, and then together generate alternative explanations to provide better understanding.

Evaluating the advantages and disadvantages of the patient's coping responses: The aim is to make patients notice that the schemas would have been once the key components for survival sometime during their lifetime but not anymore.

Conducting dialogues between the "schema side" and the "healthy side": Adapted from the "empty chair technique" of Gestalt therapy, the therapist guides the patient to produce healthy answers to the "schema side" and then they switch places and the client plays the "healthy side" or plays both the "healthy side" and the "schema side" and generates healthy answers to accusations of the schema.

Schema flash cards: Patients carry these coping cards when their schemas get activated.

Schema diary: Patients use these diaries again when their schemas are triggered. They identify the triggering event, emotions, thoughts, schema underneath, realistic and unrealistic concerns, and the healthy responses to these.

Following the cognitive strategies, experiential change strategies which include reparenting (imaginary dialogues between the vulnerable child, unhealthy adult, and the healthy adult) take place, letters to the parent and imagination for pattern-breaking [31].

Schema therapy of ASPD is a long journey with obstacles requiring the motivation of both the patient and the therapist. During the process, the therapist must prepare himself/herself for the therapy interfering behaviors/obstacles such as schema avoidance-detached protector mode, anger control problems, alcohol/substance abuse, and criminal behaviors/legal issues and keep his/her own schemas, avoidances, and overcompensations as well.

3. Conclusion

In conclusion, antisocial personality disorder has a great burden on the society in terms of both the financial expenses to treat the disorder and the juridical problems. Yet, there are no satisfactory results in the treatment of ASPD. Full (optimal) remission seems to be an unrealistic target for health professionals. The biggest obstacle is the demotivation of the client, which results in disengagement to the therapy or even not attending the sessions properly. It would not be surprising for the client to commit therapy interfering behaviors like cheating, lying, or even ridiculing the therapist. Cognitive behavioral-oriented therapies hypothesize that antisocial persons see themselves as unlovable, lonely, etc., which may be a compensation of victimization and suggest focusing on cognitive restructuring of the intermediate beliefs. Although there is not enough evidence of any psychotherapeutic interventions that are significantly effective, improvements in the symptoms like impulsivity, aggressive behaviour, or substance misuse will definitely have positive effects not only on the society in general (like reducing crime rates, etc.) but also on the interpersonal relations that the client have with the others.

Author details

Ahmet Emre Sargın[1]*, Kadir Özdel[2] and Mehmet Hakan Türkçapar[3]

*Address all correspondence to: esargin79@yahoo.com

1 Department of Psychology, Uskudar University, Istanbul, Turkey

2 Dışkapı Yıldırım Beyazıt Training and Research Hospital, Ankara, Turkey

3 Department of Psychology, Hasan Kalyoncu University, Gaziantep, Turkey

References

[1] American Psychiatric Association. Diagnostic and Statistical Manual of Mental Disorders. 4th ed. Washington, DC: American Psychiatric Publishing; 1994

[2] Dinwiddie SH, Daw EW. Temporal stability of antisocial personality disorder: Blind follow-up study at 8 years. Comprehensive Psychiatry. 1998;**39**(1):29-34

[3] De Ruiter C, Greeven PG. Personality disorders in a Dutch forensic psychiatric sample: Convergence of interview and self-report measures. Journal of Personality Disorders. 2000;(14):162-170

[4] American Psychiatric Association. Diagnostic and Statistical Manual for Mental Disorders. 5th ed. Washington, DC: American Psychiatric Publishing; 2013

[5] Swanson MC, Bland RC, Newman SC. Epidemiology of psychiatric disorders in Edmonton. Antisocial personality disorders. Acta Psychiatrica Scandinavica, Supplementum. 1994; **376**:63-70

[6] Ozarin L. Moral insanity: A brief history. Psychiatric News. 2001;**36**(10):21

[7] Cleckley H. The Mask of Sanity. 1st ed. St. Louis: Mosby; 1941

[8] Hare RD. The Hare Psychopathy Checklist-Revised (PCL-R). 2nd ed. Toronto, Canada: Multi-health Systems; 2003

[9] Lilienfeld S. Conceptual problems in the assessment of psychopathy. Clinical Psychology Review. 1994;**14**:17-38

[10] Herpertz SC, Werth U, Lukas G, Qunaibi M, Schuerkens A, Kunert H, Freese R, Flesch M, Mueller-Isberner A, Osterheider M, et al. Emotion in criminal offenders with psychopathy and borderline personality disorder. Archives of General Psychiatry. 2001;**58**:737-745

[11] Harpur TJ, Hakstian AR, Hare RD. Factor structure of the psychopathy checklist. Journal of Consulting and Clinical Psychology. 1988;**56**:741-747

[12] Torgensen S, Kringlen E, Cramer V. The prevalence of personality disorders in a community sample. Archives of General Psychiatry. 2001;**58**:590-596

[13] Hart SD, Hare RD. Psychopathy: Assessment and association with the criminal conduct. In: Stoff DM, Breiling J, Maser JD, editors. Handbook of Antisocial Behavior. 1st ed. New York, USA: Wiley; 1997. pp. 22-35

[14] Widiger TA, Corbitt EM. Comorbidity of antisocial personality disorder with other personality disorders. In: Stoff DM, Breiling JM, Maser JD, editors. Handbook of Antisocial Behaviors. 1st ed. New York, USA: Wiley; 1997. pp. 75-82

[15] Robins LN, Tipp J, Przybeck T. Antisocial personality. In: Robins LN, Legiar DA, editors. Psychiatric Disorders in America. 1st ed. New York: Free Press; 1991. pp. 258-290

[16] Lenzenweger MF, Lane MC, Loranger AW. DSM-IV personality disorders in the National Comorbidity Survey Replication. Biological Psychiatry. 2007;**15**:553-564

[17] Cadoret RJ, Yates WR, Troughton E, Woodworth G, Stewart MA. Genetic-environmental interaction in the genesis of agressively and conduct disorders. Archives of General Psychiatry. 1995;**52**(11):916-924

[18] Eysenck HJ, Gudjonsson GH. The Causes and Cures of Criminality. 1st ed. New York, USA: Plenum; 1989

[19] Hare RD. Electrodermal and cardiovascular correlates of psychopathy. In: Hare RD, Schalling D, editors. Psychopathic Behavior: Approaches to Research. 1st ed. New York, USA: Wiley; 1978. pp. 107-143

[20] Beck AT, Freeman A. Cognitive Theory of Personality Disorders. 1st ed. New York, USA: Guilford Press; 1990

[21] Beck AT, Rush AJ, Shaw BF, Emery G. Cognitive Therapy of Depression. New York, USA: Guilford Press; 1979

[22] Beck JS. Cognitive Behavior Therapy: Basics and Beyond. New York, USA: Guilford Press; 2011

[23] Ellis A. Reason and Emotion in Psychotherapy. New York, USA: Lyle Stuart; 1962

[24] Padesky CA. Schema change processes in cognitive therapy. Clinical Psychology Psychotherapy. 1994;**1**(5):267-278

[25] Beck AT, Davis DD, Freeman A. Cognitive Therapy of Personality Disorders. 3rd ed. New York, USA: Guilford Press; 2015

[26] Hofmann SG, Fang A. The efficacy of cognitive behavioral therapy: A review of meta-analyses. Cognitive Therapy and Research. 2012;**36**:427-440

[27] Butler AC, Chapman JE, Forman EM, Beck AT. The empirical status of cognitive-behavioral therapy: A review of meta-analyses. Clinical Psychology Review. 2006;**26**:17-31

[28] Clark DA, Beck AT, Alford BA. Scientific Foundations of Cognitive Theory and Therapy of Depression. Hoboken, NJ: Wiley; 1999

[29] Clark DA, Beck AT. Cognitive Therapy of Anxiety Disorders: Science and Practice. New York, USA: Guilford Press; 2010

[30] Shadish WR, Matt GR, Navarro AM, Phillips G. The effects of psychological therapies under clinically representative conditions: A meta-analysis. Psychological Bulletin. 2000;**126**:512-529

[31] Young JE, Klosko JS, Weishaar ME. Schema Therapy: A Practitioner's Guide. New York, USA: Guilford Press; 2003

[32] Young JE, Lindemann MD. An integrative schema-focused model for personality disorders. Journal of Cognitive Psychotherapy: An International Quarterly. 1992;**6**:11-23

[33] Dadomo H, Grecucci A, Giardini I, Ugolini E, Carmelita A, Panzeri M. Schema therapy for emotional dysregulation: Theoretical implication and clinical applications. Frontiers in Psychology. 2016;**7**:1987. DOI: 10.3389/fpsyg.2016.01987

[34] Giesen-Bloo J, van Dyck R, Spinhoven P, van Tilburg W, Dirksen C, van Asselt T, et al. Outpatient psychotherapy for borderline personality disorder, randomised trial of schema-focused therapy vs transference-focused psychotherapy. Archives of General Psychiatry. 2006;**63**:649-658

[35] Farrel JM, Shaw IA, Webber AA. A schema-focused approach to group psychotherapy for outpatients with borderline personality disorder: A randomized controlled trial. Behavior Therapy and Experimental Psychiatry. 2009;**40**:317-328

[36] Dickhaut V, Arnzt A. Combined group and individual schema therapy for borderline personality disorder: A pilot study. Journal of Behavior Therapy and Experimental Psychiatry. 2014;**45**(2):242-251

[37] Bamelis LL, Evers SM, Spinhoven P, Arntz A. Results of a multicenter randomized controlled trial of the clinical effectiveness of schema therapy for personality disorders. American Journal of Psychiatry. 2014;**171**(3):305-322

[38] Jovev M, Jackson H. Early maladaptive schemas in personality disordered individuals. Journal of Personality Disorders. 2004;**18**(5):467-478

[39] Nordahl HM, Holthe H, Haugum JA. Early maladaptive schemas in patients with or without personality disorders: Does schema modification predict symptomatic relief? Clinical Psychology & Psychotherapy. 2005;**12**(2):142-149

[40] Reeves M, Taylor J. Specific relationships between core beliefs and personality disorder symptoms in a non-clinical sample. Clinical Psychology and Psychotherapy. 2007; **14**:96-104

[41] Freeman A, Pretzer J, Fleming B, Simon KM. Clinical Applications of Cognitive Therapy. New York, USA: Plenum Press; 1990

[42] Millon T, Everly G. Personality and its Disorders: A Biosocial Learning Approach. New York: Wiley; 1985

[43] Tremblay PF, Dozois DJA. Another perspective on trait aggressiveness: Overlap with early maladaptive schemas. Personality and Individual Differences. 2009;**46**:569-574

[44] Gilbert F, Daffern M, Talevski D, Ogloff JR. The role of aggression-related cognition in the agressive behaviors of offenders: A general aggression model perspective. Criminal Justice and Behavior. 2013;**40**(2):119-138

[45] Loper AB. The relationship of maladaptive beliefs to personality and behavioral adjustment among incarcerated women. Journal of Cognitive Psychotherapy. 2003; **17**(3):253-266

[46] Ward T. Sexual offenders' cognitive distortions as implicit theories. Aggression and Violent Behavior. 2000;**5**:491-507

[47] Polaschek DL, Calvert SW, Gannon TA. Linking violent thinking: Implicit theory-based research with violent offenders. Journal of Interpersonal Violence. 2009;**24**:75-96

[48] Ozdel, K, Turkcapar MH, Guriz SO, Hamamci Z, Duy B, Taymur I, et al. Early maladaptive schemas and core beliefs in antisocial personality disorder. International Journal of Cognitive Therapy. 2015;**8**(4):306-317

[49] Beck AT, Freeman A, Davis DD. Cognitive Therapy of Personality Disorders. 2nd ed. New York: Guilford Press; 2004

[50] Meloy JR, Yakeley J. Antisocial personality disorder. In: Gabbard GO, editor. Gabbard's Treatment of Psychiatric Disorders. 5th ed. Arlington. APA Publishing; 2014

[51] Gibbon S, Duggan C, Stoffers J, Huband N, Völmm BA, Ferriter M et al. Psychological interventions for antisocial personality disorder. Cochrane Database of Systematic Reviews. 2010:CD 007668

[52] Davidson KM, Tyrer P, Tata P, Cooke D, Gumley A, Ford I, et al. Cognitive behavior therapy for violent man with antisocial personality disorder in the community: An exploratory randomized controlled trial. Psychological Medicine. 2009;**39**(4):569-577

[53] Matusiewicz AK, Hopwood CJ, Banducci AN, Lejuez CW. The effectiveness of cognitive behavioral therapy for personality disorders. Psychiatric Clinics of North America. 2010;**33**(3):657-685

[54] Hoffman SG, Asnaani A, Vonk IJ, Sawyer AT, Fang A. The efficacy of cognitive behavioral therapy: A review of meta-analyses. Cognitive Therapy and Research. 2012;**36**(5): 427-440

[55] Andrews Da, Bonta J. Psychology of Criminal Conduct. 5th ed. London and New York: Routledge; 2010

[56] Andrews DA, Bonta J, Wormith JS. The recent past and near future of risk and/or need assessment. Crime & Delinquency. 2006;**52**(1):7-27

[57] Butler AC, Beck AT, Cohen LH. The personality belief questionnaire-short form: Development and preliminary findings. Cognitive Therapy and Research. 2007;**31**(3):357-370

[58] Dobson D, Dobson KS. Evidence-based Practice of Cognitive-behavioral Therapy. 2nd ed. New York: Guilford Press; 2016

[59] Alexander F, French TM. Psychoanalytic Therapy: Principles and Applications. New York: Ronald Press; 1946

Chapter 6

Psychopathy: A Behavioral Systems Approach

Liane J. Leedom

Additional information is available at the end of the chapter

http://dx.doi.org/10.5772/intechopen.69488

Abstract

Why do they do that? is the question theories of psychopathy should answer. Current theories of psychopathy fail to answer this question because they focus on affective and inhibitory deficits rather than on motivation. Antisocial behavior is appetitive and therefore can only be explained with a motivational theory. This chapter presents a motivational theory of psychopathy that draws on the ethological framework. The chapter answers all four questions of ethology as applied to psychopathy.

Keywords: psychopathy, love, attachment, caregiving, dominance, behavioral systems

1. Introduction

Why do they do that? is the question most frequently asked by those whose lives have been touched by someone with psychopathy. The "that" in the question refers to a myriad of harm inflicting and gratuitously destructive behaviors such as: pathological lying; conning; manipulation; psychological, social, financial, physical and sexual abuse; thievery; and squandering of financial resources and possessions. Although those without psychopathy also sporadically engage in harmful behaviors, these behaviors constitute raison d'être for the psychopathic. To date theories of psychopathy that focus on deficits in social emotions and impulse control have failed to explain "why they do that" [1–3]. The fallacious assumption of "deficit" theories is that were it not for inhibitory mechanisms, all people would be antisocial. As a psychiatrist trained in the methods of ethology, I reject: (1) the idea that deficits "cause" behavior and (2) that all people are motivated to be antisocial. Instead, I propose that specific motivational systems are affected by psychopathy and that these affected systems cause antisocial behavior at all levels of the disorder. While I do not dispute that dysregulation of motives is part of psychopathy, lack of inhibition alone does not explain the behavioral syndrome. Understanding "why they do that" begins with understanding motives and motivational systems. As psychologist Partridge [4], said nearly 90 years ago, "These persons display, first of all, persistent and chronic sociopathic behavior. This chronic behavior, to be regarded as essentially sociopathic, is to be understandably related in some way to their motivations with respect to their major interests and urges." This chapter presents an ethologically-based motivational theory of psychopathy that explains the manifest behavior of psychopathic individuals and addresses all four of the central questions of ethology. The theory is ethologically based due to my early training and because the discipline of ethology seeks to answer the "why, what and how questions" of behavior. I begin by briefly outlining the four questions and epistemic roots of ethology.

2. The ethological approach[1]

The first question of ethology is "why do these animals behave as they do [8]?" To explore this first question ethologists make extensive naturalistic observations and create thorough descriptions of behavior prior to any experimental study. In ethology, induction precedes deduction. Ethologists also place observational and experimental data into a developmental and an evolutionary framework. How did the behavior develop? What is its function? and What is its phylogeny? are questions 2–4 of ethology [8, 9]. In asking these questions ethologists maintain that any complete explanation of behavior should address proximate causation in terms of stimulus response mechanisms and development, and ultimate causation in terms of function and phylogeny [8]. Extensive observations of the naturalistic behavior of vertebrates including primates led to the discovery of behavioral systems that operate similarly to other biological adaptive control systems. Behavioral systems govern "the motivation and control of a group of behavior patterns that are closely and more or less causally (and often also functionally) related to each other [10]." Hence, goal directed behaviors important to survival and reproduction are the output of particular adaptive control systems. The existence of behavioral systems may be inferred from output behaviors and then the physiological mechanisms that comprise the system may be studied. Three processes define adaptive control systems: continuous monitoring (by sensors), comparison between actual state and desired state (by comparators), and output to achieve the desired state (by enactors). Studies of behavioral systems determine salient stimuli, examine correlates of goal states (in terms of internal working models), and describe physiological and behavioral outputs of the system. It is behavioral systems that organize information processing, and govern the choice, activation and termination of behavioral sequences.

[1]Why do not motives figure more prominently in theories of psychopathy? In 1973 the Nobel Prize in Physiology or Medicine was awarded jointly to ethologists Karl von Frisch, Konrad Lorenz and Nikolaas Tinbergen "for their discoveries concerning organization and elicitation of individual and social behavior patterns [5]." Subsequently, sociological forces led to the decline of the influence of ethology on clinicians and researchers. In the decades that followed, the Nazi past of Lorenz was exposed, and sociobiology and comparative psychology arose as replacements for the discipline forever tainted by one of its founders [6]. The science of motivation also waned due to the demise of drive theory as conceived of by Freud and Lorenz [7]. Although there were good reasons for the demise of ethology; loss of the methods and ideas of this discipline has negatively impacted understanding of both normative and pathological human behavior.

2.1. Four human social behavioral systems

In humans, social behavior and the learning of social behavior is mediated through four innate behavioral systems: the attachment/affiliation, care-giving, dominance and sexual systems. These systems serve the adaptive goals of: safety through affiliation, parental care, competition (dominance/resource control) and mating. These systems are innate but important maturational experiences guide their normative development. (For a complete discussion of human social behavioral systems see Ref. [11].) Although all four human social behavioral systems contribute to behavioral disorders [11–13] only the attachment/affiliation system is recognized widely by clinicians due to the work of Bowlby [14, 15]. Bowlby, a psychoanalyst was strongly influenced by ethologist Robert Hinde [16].

2.1.1. Significance and salience acquisition and salience attribution to others

Reinforcement processes operate through the brain reward system to reify the behavioral strategies of the social behavioral systems [11]. Research on addiction has provided much insight into the psychobiology of reward and therefore social behavioral systems. Behaviors enacted in goal acquisition are reinforced, and rewarding stimuli are primary reinforcers. Just as tasty food is reinforcing through the feeding system, contact comfort, dependent stimuli, others' submissive responses and sexual contact are reinforcing through the attachment, caregiving, dominance and sexual systems. Situational stimuli signal the presence of primary rewards and these stimuli acquire incentive salience. Attribution of incentive salience differs between individuals and this individual difference confers risk for addictive disorders [17]. Furthermore salience attribution is impaired by addiction [18].

The process of special significance and salience acquisition and subsequent attribution of salience to others within the social behavioral systems is called "bonding" [19]. Individuals who are the source of attachment reward acquire special significance and are attributed salience in development [19]. Similarly salience is attributed to individuals who are the objects of care [20], and to mates [21]. Whether individuals associated with dominance reward acquire special significance and salience has not been investigated (though the existence of slavery suggests some form of social tie to the subjugated). Bonding to a caregiver early in life appears to affect the process of special significance and salience acquisition such that failure to establish an attachment bond is associated with failure to give care to offspring, failure to bond to mates and to risk for addiction (for detailed discussion see Ref. [11]).

2.1.2. Love

The terms bond, attachment and love have been used interchangeably in the literature however, I contend that the word "love" should be used to only to signify an affiliative bond that also involves caregiving. The term attachment should be used to reflect the tendency to seek proximity to another in times of need (for security). According to Shaver and Mikulincer [22] romantic love should be conceptualized in terms of the activity of three interdependent behavioral systems—attachment, caregiving and sex. This definition provides a framework for investigating love in those with high levels of psychopathic traits as the attachment (ABS), caregiving (CGS) and sexual (SBS) behavioral systems, as well as the interrelationships them can be examined. Inherent within this framework is the idea that behavioral systems are subject to activation and deactivation and may inhibit or stimulate one another as neural networks are simultaneously activated or deactivated.

The behavioral and neurobiological integration of the social behavioral systems is complex and therefore subject to individual variation and disorder. One developmental task of childhood is to integrate the attachment, dominance and caregiving systems, with the integration of the sexual system occurring in adolescence [11]. Successful development and integration of the attachment, caregiving and sexual systems determines an individual's capacity for deep intimate relationships and committed romantic love. This integration occurs at both a neural-physiological and a behavioral level. When a man or woman "falls in love" with a romantic partner, sexual arousal and the resultant neuroendocrine sequelae give rise to a love bond. The caregiving behavioral system is subsequently activated by communications of need by the loved one. Capacity for love is linked to the effective functioning of the caregiving behavioral system and the degree to which the three systems integrate. Other love relationships are likened to romantic love as they share a common neurobiological mechanism—the activity of the attachment and caregiving behavioral systems.

3. Psychopathy and love

Maslow in his classic paper, A theory of human motivation, declared, "The so-called 'psychopathic personality' is another example of permanent loss of the love needs. These are people who, according to the best data available, have been starved for love in the earliest months of their lives and have simply lost forever the desire and the ability to give and to receive affection (as animals lose sucking or pecking reflexes that are not exercised soon enough after birth) [23]." (Note that this loss of the capacity for love was theoretically linked to early developmental experiences and love is equated with affection.) Contemporaneously with Maslow, Cleckley described psychopathic individuals in The Mask of Sanity and developed a set of criteria for their identification. According to Cleckley (criteria #9), psychopathy is associated with "pathological egocentricity and incapacity for love." He stated (p. 347), "The psychopath [sic][2] seldom shows anything that, **if the chief facts were known**, would pass even in the eyes of lay observers as object love (emphasis added)." Why Cleckley connected pathological egocentricity with incapacity for love is not explained in his writing. It is also not immediately apparent what Cleckley meant when he used the word "love" in his criteria. It seems that even he struggled with its definition:

In a sense, it is absurd to maintain that the psychopath's [sic] incapacity for object love is absolute, that is, to say he is (in)capable of affection for another … He is plainly capable of casual fondness, of likes and dislikes, and of reactions that, one might say, cause others to matter to him. These affective reactions

[2]It is against ethical guidelines to refer to a person by his/her diagnosis. The author hopes that others will join in not using the term "psychopath" in scientific discourse. This term is also misleading in that it implies categorical status for this construct.

are, however, always strictly limited in degree. In durability they also vary greatly from what is normal in mankind. The term absolute is, I believe, appropriate if we apply it to any affective attitude strong and meaningful enough to be called love, that is, anything that prevails in sufficient degree and over sufficient periods to exert a major influence on behavior (p. 347).

Important to dimensional diagnosis, Cleckley also maintained that an "absolute" incapacity for love is found even in those with an "incomplete manifestation" of psychopathy, who lack the full disorder. Kernberg [24] connected incapacity for love to egocentricity by suggesting that pathological narcissism is the foundation or core of psychopathy. Indeed, many characteristics of pathological narcissism are features of psychopathy, including egocentricity, grandiosity, low empathy, a sense of entitlement, interpersonal exploitativeness, dominance and aggression, hostility and antagonism. Writing in 1956, McCord and McCord disagreed with Cleckley and Maslow. They described psychopathic persons as having "a warped capacity for love" stating, "there are indications that the capacity, however under developed, still exists [25]."

Today many still assume, "psychopaths [sic] are characterized by an inability to form lasting bonds [26]." Lack of bonds is thought to be connected to lack of love, or deficient social emotions. The DSM 5 committee proposed the following prototype description for antisocial/psychopathic personality disorder: "Their emotional expression is mostly limited to irritability, anger, and hostility; *acknowledgement and articulation of other emotions, such as love or anxiety, are rare* (italics added) [27]." Although withdrawn, this prototype description reflects both historical perspectives and a failure to give credence to the many naturalistic observations of psychopathic individuals that appear in the literature. A review of case histories [28–31], research accounts of family members [30], and journalist biographies [32] reveals that many psychopathic individuals do in fact maintain social ties[3] over extended years. They often profess love for children and other family members. It is therefore imperative to explain rather than deny social ties, and expressions of affection in psychopathic individuals.

In a unique study, Gawda [33] examined "love scripts" in prisoners with and without the diagnosis of antisocial personality disorder (ASPD). She asked subjects to look at a photograph of a couple hugging each other and to "Imagine you are one of the people in the photograph. Try to identify with your role. Write a story about it." Those diagnosed with ASPD wrote significantly longer stories than prisoners not diagnosed, but their stories were similar in length to those of non-prisoners. Their stories also described more actors' traits, strong emotions, presumptions, wishes and self-concentration. Contrary to the proposed DSM prototype, prisoners with ASPD were able to acknowledge and articulate "love" when asked to. This data is consistent with the glibness and superficial charm that may characterize these individuals. It also shows that this group possesses cognitive schema for "love." Other evidence that antisocial individuals possess knowledge of and articulate love comes from our internet survey of spouses, romantic partners and family member of putative psychopathic individuals. Only a minority of those surveyed reported the individual rarely articulated

[3]I agree that highly psychopathic individuals are incapable of love; the term "bond" is associated with the term love. Therefore I use the phrase "social ties" to describe the social bonds psychopathic individuals have with family members and friends. The loss of significant relationships may evoke distress in psychopathic persons.

love. When asked to describe in an open ended format the love behavior, many spouses and romantic partners reported being "love bombed" or lavished with attention, affirmations of love and gifts early in the relationship [34].

In a recent paper, myself and colleagues [30] detailed (among other cases) the case of German national Christian Karl Gerhartsreiter, AKA "Clark Rockefeller," a psychopathic (traits described by forensic evaluators) con artist and convicted murderer who charmed financial executive Sandra Boss. They married and resided together for 12 years. He fathered then kidnapped their 9 year old child when Ms. Boss divorced him (after discovering the deception). While on trial for kidnapping he stated, regarding Ms. Boss, "I absolutely love her; I wish she hadn't walked out on me." Regarding their daughter he stated, "I just want to be a father. I just want to be with her, I want to get her up in the morning, send her off to school, walk her to the bus, wait when she comes back and give her something to eat at night and put her back to bed then the same again." These statements made in court were so convincing that the judge said, "The defendant was by all accounts a loving and devoted father to his daughter." I mention this case as an example of the many observations that refute the notion that psychopathic individuals (as defined by DSM, Cleckley and PCL-R criteria) do not form lasting social ties or "articulate love." According to romantic partner and family member accounts, psychopathic individuals often vociferously proclaim love for family members; and as in the case above, psychopathic individuals may display caring behaviors (possibly as part of a presentation management strategy) and so appear loving [34].

The misconception that psychopathic individuals do not express love or form lasting social ties could result in inexperienced clinicians or those trying to strictly apply an erroneous prototype, being misled and missing the diagnosis of psychopathic personality. Because of the high prevalence of this personality type in domestic violence cases [35] and the problems partners have had protecting children from psychopathic parents [30], it is imperative that this misconception be addressed and the nature of social ties in psychopathic persons clarified. While I do agree that psychopathy is connected to an incapacity for love, determining this incapacity may be practically difficult due to behaviors associated with the dominance behavioral system (see below). Insomuch as capacity for love depends on the attachment and caregiving behavioral systems, it follows that either one or both of these is affected by psychopathy.

3.1. Psychopathy and the attachment behavioral system

A number of recent studies have examined the construct of psychopathy from the perspective of the Five Factor Model. Psychopathy entails reduced scores in five facets of agreeableness (straightforwardness, altruism, compliance, modesty, tender mindedness; three facets of conscientiousness (dutifulness, self-discipline, and deliberation); and one facet each of neuroticism (self-consciousness) and extraversion (warmth); and elevated scores in impulsiveness from neuroticism and excitement seeking from extraversion [36]. There exists considerable data regarding the relationship between these traits and aspects of the scientifically validated working definition of love described herein. The Five Factor Model thus generates predicted relationships between attachment and the psychopathic personality pattern. Given their characteristically low levels of agreeableness and high levels of interpersonal antagonism such adults would be expected to display a dismissive or avoidant attachment style and obtain low pleasure from closeness. However, some psychopathic individuals characteristically have positive emotions, low anxiety and are prone to excitement seeking (activation of the exploration system), all these features are associated with secure attachment in adults. Psychopathic individuals may also be quite sociable related to agenic extraversion and dominance, again traits statistically linked to secure attachment. Therefore, lack of pleasure in closeness or the dismissive/avoidant style may not be apparent on casual observation or self-report. Psychopathic individuals who enjoy dominating and manipulating others may even find social interactions quite enjoyable and therefore display charm and positive affect. Relationships based on sexual gratification may also bring them pleasure. There is a subset of psychopathic individuals who are particularly prone to the negative emotions anger and anxiety [37]. These individuals may display insecure forms of attachment. Although statistically lack of secure attachment is associated with low self-esteem and low social self-efficacy, "insecurity" in psychopathic individuals has different correlates. It links to egocentrism, unstable self-esteem, entitlement and a desire to maintain power and status in the face of uncertainty in being able to do so [38].

Temperament and Character Inventory (TCI) Novelty Seeking is related to Big Five excitement seeking and tends to be elevated in antisocial individuals; this trait has a weak relationship to attachment anxiety and no relationship to avoidant attachment. TCI Reward Dependence is a measure of the rewarding properties of relationships. Reward Dependence is low in antisocial individuals; and low reward dependence, like low agreeableness is weakly related to avoidant attachment. TCI harm avoidance is low in antisocial individuals and high in anxious individuals, and is moderately strongly related to anxious attachment [39]. In summary, personality traits studies suggest that psychopathic personality may not be strongly associated with any particular attachment style.

Interestingly, some psychopathic people are classified as attachment secure in their romantic relationships. Using the Levenson Self-Report Psychopathy Scale, one study found that primary psychopathy positively predicted greater intimacy, passion and commitment as measured by the Triangular Love Scale [40]. In this and other studies, secondary psychopathy (equivalent to high PCL-R Factor 2 scores) predicted abusive behavior and relationship dissatisfaction [41]. Using the self-report Psychopathic Personality Inventory (PPI), Dindo and Fowles found primary psychopathy to be significantly positively associated with the "social closeness" component of the Multidimensional Personality Questionnaire (MPQ) [41]. High scorers on this scale describe themselves as: sociable, liking to be with people; taking pleasure in and valuing close personal ties; warm and affectionate; turning to others for comfort and help. In contrast to PPI Factor 1, PPI Factor 2 was negatively associated with "social closeness." Another study also found PPI total scores to be unrelated to attachment insecurity [42].

Psychopathic individuals can differ with respect to PCL-R Factor 1 and Factor 2 symptoms, individuals with more Factor 1 and fewer Factor 2 symptoms may appear "securely attached" due to the presence of charm, positive emotions and social skills. One study examined the four PCL-R interpersonal/affective features most predictive of psychopathy (callousness/lack of empathy, glibness/superficial charm, lack of remorse/guilt and shallow affect) as correlated with self-reported interpersonal behavior. Psychopathic individuals reported less self-directed hostility (less harsh introjects) and perceived significant others to withdraw less even during arguments [43]. In support of a lack of association between psychopathy and insecure attachment, Brennen and Shaver found a lack of association between self-reported attachment style and a Personality Disorder Questionnaire Factor they labeled "psychopathy" [44].

Consistent with the importance of high Factor 2 scores in predicting attachment insecurity, psychopathic personality is more clearly associated with avoidant or dismissive attachment in criminal populations. Offenders, irrespective of the degree of psychopathy are likely to show less secure attachment, report more instability in relationships, less emotional attachment to others, and a strong wish for personal autonomy. Violent offenders are by no means all insecurely attached [45]. Both Frodi et al. [46] and van IJzendoorn et al. [47] found that secure attachment (assessed by the Adult Attachment Interview [AAI]) did exist but was uncommon among personality disordered criminal offenders. These studies in addition to that of Rosenstein and Horowitz [48] point to an overrepresentation of avoidant attachment representations among individuals with 'externalizing' problems (again consistent with an association between Factor 2 and insecure attachment). Brody and Rosenfeld [26] examined object relations in psychopathic offenders also finding that insecure attachment was significantly correlated with Total PCL:SV and Factor 2 scores but not with scores on Factor 1.

Given that the research linking attachment with antisocial/psychopathic personality seems inconsistent, it is curious that the disorder has been so strongly connected to a lack of love [49, 50]. According to behavioral systems theory, love involves caregiving (and sometimes sex) in addition to attachment. Furthermore, social reward and resultant positive affect may also be obtained from dominating others. The next sections reveal that the data regarding the involvement of the caregiving, dominance and sexual systems in psychopathy is stronger than that implicating the attachment system. That a "parasitic lifestyle" is a symptom of psychopathy speaks against psychopathy being associated with an inability to get material needs met through relationships (the goal of the attachment behavioral system). Clearly psychopathic individuals do seek social ties for that purpose.

3.2. Psychopathy and the caregiving behavioral system

There is strong support for the idea that psychopathy is associated with impairment in the caregiving behavioral system (CGS). Empathy, which is critical to CGS working models is impaired by psychopathy [51]. Impaired empathy (callousness) is diagnostic of psychopathy and failure to care for children is a DSM IIIR diagnostic criteria for antisocial personality disorder [52]. The Big Five personality traits associated with psychopathy are those associated with low warmth toward children, authoritarian (dominating) and neglectful parenting. One study assessed mothering by interview and observation in a group of women diagnosed as antisocial through Minnesota Multiphasic Personality Inventory-2 (MMPI-2) profiles [53]. Antisocial mothers showed lack of warmth, passivity/neglect, harsh/abusive discipline, inconsistent/ineffective discipline, poor monitoring and supervision, and possessed aggressive values. Another study assessed psychopathy and attachment patterns in relation to maternal behavior in incarcerated female offenders. Psychopathy correlated with dismissive attachment patterns in women and higher rates of voluntary relinquishment of young children [54]. With respect to fathers, Kirkman [55] interviewed partners of psychopathic men. These partners reported the men psychologically abused children by: "(1) lying to them; (2) ignoring them; (3) failing to provide for them; (4) bullying and terrifying them; (5) breaking promises to them; (and) (6) destroying their toys." I have found that psychopathic parents do give care to children and support them financially; however, this care is often inconsistent and out of sink with the needs of the child [30]. Psychopathic parents do seek custody of children through the family courts often to exact revenge on a former partner or to avoid financial loss or responsibility. Psychopathic parents may also choose "favorites" and "targets" from among the children of the family; targets are rejected and abused while favorites are overindulged in a manner that serves the needs of the psychopathic parent. These aberrant parenting behaviors reflect lack of caregiving internal working models, low sensitivity and responsiveness derived from lack of empathy, as well as low warmth which may be associated with little pleasure in intimacy. Given the deficits in the CGS, it is remarkable that psychopathic persons function as parents at all. As discussed below, caregiving behaviors may serve power goals and so also reflect dominance motives. The dominance behavioral system enacts coercive control, harsh/abusive discipline, aggressive values, lying, and other aggressive acts.

One recent study examined impaired empathy in male perpetrators of intimate partner violence and its relationship to psychopathic traits as measured by the Self-Report Psychopathy Scale [56]. Psychopathy scores were significantly correlated with impaired perceptions of wife and other female expressions of both happiness and fear. Expressions of happiness may actually trigger aggression due to happiness being misinterpreted as disgust. There was a positive relationship between psychopathy and the perpetration of intimate partner violence; however this relationship was only weakly mediated by impaired emotion recognition. These results support the contention that impaired empathy alone does not explain aggression. Impaired empathy is not specific to antisocial disorders. The apathetic responses toward others' distress in individuals with autism spectrum disorders (ASDs) contrast with the aggressive responses toward others' distress seen in those with antisocial disorders. Hence, it appears that both ASDs and antisocial disorders involve disruption in social reward, empathy and the CGS. However, only antisocial individuals are characteristically manipulative and instrumentally aggressive. These observations speak against deficits in empathy as directly causal to aggressive interpersonal behavior. Instead a specific motive linked to activation of the dominance system is likely causal to antisocial behavior [57] as discussed in the following section.

4. Psychopathy and the dominance behavioral system

Clinical observations and numerous studies link DBS functioning to psychopathy. Non-verbal dominance behavior including making eye contact with the interviewer, using hand gestures, leaning forward and diminished smiling is common in psychopathic individuals [58, 59]. Bursten [60] described the power motivation of the psychopathic individuals in his clinical practice as follows: "the intention to *influence the other* by employing a deception of some sort, and the *feeling of exhilaration* at having put something over on the other person if the deception is successful…The manipulative personality……is driven to manipulate primarily by his inner dynamic position...He will *seek out situations* where he can manipulate and will tend to provoke conflict in goals in order to set the stage for his manipulation [60]." In the only empirical study of power motivation, delinquent girls were found to have elevated levels [61].

In a study examining responses to the semi-projective interviewer administered Sentence Completion Test (SCT) in a group of offenders, PCL-R psychopathy correlated with an ego-centric, manipulative interpersonal orientation, increased ideation regarding possessing power and dominating others, and reactance. Power concern and the use of profanity formed a factor which was not specific for high PCL-R scores. However, the factor was very *sensitive for the absence of PCL-R psychopathy* in that "if a subject did not manifest the indicators of psychopathy in the SCT, he was almost certainly not a psychopath [sic] [62]."

Dominance behavior is diagnostic of psychopathy. The interpersonal facet items of the PCL-R: glibness and superficial charm, grandiose sense of self-worth, pathological lying, and cunning/manipulative behavior comprise a dominance style that is typical of psychopathy. This psychopathy-related bi-strategic dominance style is adaptive in that it enables individuals to attract and extract positive investment from others including friends, extended family, children and potential mates [28, 31, 31, 34]. Klein [63] explained why pathological lying signals dominance motivation stating, "Above all every deception, every imposture is an assumption of power. The person deceived is reduced in stature, symbolically nullified, while the imposture is temporarily powerful, even greater than if he were the real thing." At least three Comprehensive Assessment of Psychopathic Personality-Institutional Rating Scale (CAPP-IRS) domains index the DBS: the dominance domain (domineering, deceitful, manipulative, insincere, garrulous), the self-domain (self-centered, self-aggrandizing, sense of uniqueness, sense of entitlement, sense of invulnerability, self-justify) and the behavioral domain (aggressive, disruptive). In answering the question, "What is a Psychopath [sic]?" experts and lay people in the United States and Europe [64–67] consistently rate the self and dominance domains as prototypical of psychopathy.

The Interpersonal Measure of Psychopathy developed by Kosson and colleagues [68] assesses, alliance seeking, expressed narcissism, showmanship and the degree to which the subject incorporates the interviewer into stories. Each of these reflects ingratiating or relatively "prosocial" dominance strategies. IM-P total scores correlate significantly with PCL-R total, Factor 1, and Factor 2 [68–70]. IM-P total scores also correlate with IASR-B5 observer-rated and self-rated dominance [68, 70]. Due to dominant interpersonal behavior, psychopathy maps into quadrant 2 of interpersonal circumplex space as assessed by both observational (CIRCLE) and self-report measures (IAS, IASR-B5 and IIP). Individuals placed in the mid-section of quadrant 2 are: arrogant, manipulative, cynical, exhibitionistic, sensation-seeking, Machiavellian, and vindictive [71].

Instrumental aggression is hurtful behavior directed toward achieving power through intimidation and subjugation. In an extensive literature, psychopathy, is associated with instrumental, reactive, relational and laboratory aggression [72–75]. Factor 1 correlates with these more than does Factor 2, except for reactive aggression [74]. Instrumental aggression is more strongly associated with psychopathy than is reactive aggression [75]. Psychopathy also predicts the use of social aggression in mating competition [76]. The next section describes the sexual behavioral system and link this system to manifestations of psychopathy.

5. Psychopathy and the sexual behavioral system

A discussion of the relationship between sociosexuality[4] and individual differences in general personality traits is pertinent to this discussion as is the relationship between psychopathy and sociosexual orientation. Sensation seeking, low agreeableness and low conscientiousness are linked to psychopathic personality and these traits are associated with less restricted sociosexual orientation. As part of the International Sexuality Description Project, 13,243 participants from 46 nations responded to self-report measures of personality and sexuality [77]. Several traits showed consistent links with unrestricted sociosexuality. Extraversion was universally associated with unrestricted sociosexuality, having engaged in short-term mate poaching attempts, having succumbed to short-term poaching attempts, and lacking relationship exclusivity. Studies have also linked impulsive sensation-seeking to short-term mating [78], including men's patronage of prostitutes [79]. Impulsive sensation-seeking is closely associated with the Big Five dimensions of low agreeableness and low conscientiousness [80, 81]. Not surprisingly, low agreeableness and low conscientiousness have been linked directly short-term mating, especially with measures of extra-pair mating (i.e., succumbing to short-term poaching attempts) [82].

Self-Reported Psychopathy Scale scores significantly correlate with the adoption of a ludus or game playing love style, with participants endorsing items such as "I enjoy playing the 'game of love' with a number of different partners." [83, 84]. Outcalt [85] examined the relationship between ludus love style, attachment (as rated by the Experiences in Close Relationship Scale [ECR]), psychopathy (as rated by the PPI), impulsivity (as measured by the Barratt Impulsiveness Scale) and the tendency to seek social reward (as measured by the Social Errors Scale). The relationship between ludus love and psychopathy was mediated by both attachment avoidance and the tendency to seek social reward. Harris et al. [86] have identified five variables reflecting early, frequent, and coercive sex that associate strongly with psychopathy. Promiscuous sex is also a symptom of psychopathy on the PCL-R, thus research clearly links psychopathy with impersonal sexual behavior. When this approach to sex is combined with aberrant dominance motives, sexual coercion may result.

6. Why do they do that?

Cleckley [28] observed that indeed psychopathic individuals do articulate love in the service of the relationships that meet their needs. He also emphasized the lack of caregiving in psychopathic individuals pointing to an "absolute indifference to the financial, social, emotional, physical, and other hardships which he brings on those for whom he professes love." That these relationships can last over periods of years supports the idea that caregiving rather than "attachment" is primarily affected by psychopathy. This might partly explain why psychopathic individuals possess love schema and can discuss the emotion convincingly—although they do not take care of others, many have been cared for and so understand the concept.

[4]Sociosexuality indexes a person's willingness to engage in uncommitted sex.

Psychopathic individuals do rely on their social ties for at least material support, as evidenced by their parasitic lifestyles; however they are not characteristically the passive, submissive, recipients of care described in reference to attachment and the emotion Japanese label amae [87]. Since affective labels may correspond to the activity of neuronal networks, it follows that psychopathic individuals may label their hedonic experience of getting what they want (successful domination), receiving care, or sexual arousal, "love." It is reasonable to investigate this possibility rather than to assume that psychopathic individuals lack feelings and are lying or confabulating when they use the word love.

The interpersonal symptoms of psychopathy connect to the bi-strategic dominance strategies psychopathic persons employ. Superficial charm, grandiosity, pathological lying, manipulation and abuse are caused by dominance motives and an excessive need for power. The lack of a functioning caregiving system may contribute to this excessive dominance. Psychopathic individuals who lack caring motives only experience arousal of neediness (attachment), dominance (power) and/or sexual motives in the presence of others. Neediness results in parasitism; dominance and sexual motives ultimately result in abusive behavior.

Examination of the normative human personality traits connected to the social behavioral systems reveals a consistent pattern that explains the phenomenology of psychopathic personality. Individuals who are low in agreeableness (high in antagonism) and high in dysinhibition tend to have insecure attachment, deficient caregiving, high dominance and unrestricted sociosexual orientation. It is important to note that psychopathic individuals do have social motivation and may also delight in interacting with others. However, this delight stems from dominance and/or sexual reward as opposed to "love" as defined herein. Although attachment patterns are not uniform in those affected with psychopathy, when the behavioral systems definition of love is applied, psychopathy is associated with profound deficits in ability to love. These deficits stem from self-focus and what appears to be an absence of the caregiving system.

Although psychopathic individuals maintain social ties over periods of years, bonding is clearly impaired in psychopathy. Defects in significance and salience acquisition and salience attribution may causally relate to lack of bonding. These defects may link psychopathy to the addictive disorders which are prevalent in this population. Impaired salience attribution in psychopathy may also explain another curious finding—the gratuitous squandering of possessions and resources. Cleckley puzzled over this self-destructive behavior, "the psychopath [sic] often makes little or no use of what he attains as a result of deeds that eventually bring him to disaster (p. 320) (see also van den Bos et al. [88])." Psychopathy appears to impair both caring for other people and caring for possessions.

7. How does psychopathy develop?

The ethological framework allows for generation of hypotheses regarding the development of psychopathy. All four social behavioral systems are inborn; however their maturation depends on developmental experiences. The ABS begins to develop in the first year of life in a manner dependent on responsive caregiving. The CGS and empathy begin to develop shortly after the first year of life. The DBS does not normatively develop until after the second year of life. This important development sequence first noted by Harlow allows for attachment and caregiving bonds to regulate the DBS. Inhibition of dominance motivation, behavior and endocrine responses is one of the functions of love [89]. If either genetic endowment or maturational experiences affect the development of the ABS and CGS, then the result will be excessive dominance motivation and aberrant development of the DBS and SBS. Children incapable of love will be unmotivated to regulate dominance strivings and develop aggressive dominance strategies and perhaps endocrine responses that promote aggression [12] and unrestricted sociosexual orientation. Genetic endowment may also directly increase dominance motivation. An excessive need for power may subsequently erode the CGS caregiving behavioral and physiological responses.

8. What is the (adaptive) function of psychopathy?

Psychopathy may be an adaptive life-strategy of short-term mating and cheating [90, 91]. This strategy entails conceiving or birthing offspring that others care for. Psychopathic individuals thus invest energy in mating effort rather than in nurturing offspring. This strategy is only viable because most other humans are strongly motivated to care for young, even those who are not their own. Psychopathy then can be conceptualized as resulting from human cooperative breeding [92]. In cooperatively breeding species, dominant members of the group produce offspring that are cared for by other group members. Caregiving motivation is high in all non-dominant members of the group. That this strategy is more viable for men than women may account for the higher prevalence of psychopathy in men.

Another possibility is that psychopathy is not an adaptation and actually has no function and is maladaptive [93]. Psychopathy may simply be a bi-product of strong selection for social dominance [94] or lack of caregiving adaptations in some humans (see next section). Selection for social dominance would also account for higher prevalence of psychopathy in men. Across vertebrates, there is a trade-off between mating effort and caregiving such that the physiological responses that favor dominance and mating effort, suppress caregiving [95]. That psychopathy is commonly found in political leaders is evidence for the bi-product of dominance theory. Most psychopathic individuals are excessively destructive to their own families and to society; their aggression is greater than that required to ensure parasitism and that others care for their offspring. These observations suggest that while dominant behavior is an adaptation, psychopathy itself is a disorder and not an adaptation. If psychopathy is the result of cooperative breeding, and it is a disorder, it is a disorder of human society and not only of individuals.

9. What is the phylogeny of psychopathy?

Although other Hominoidea pair-bond, humans are the only cooperatively breeding species. The monogamous apes live as pairs with juvenile offspring and not in a multi-male, multi-female society. Chimpanzee society is promiscuous multi-male, multi-female and is shaped by attachment and dominance relations but not by caregiving relationships. Chimpanzees are highly aggressive and can be infanticidal [96]. Males have been observed to kill both alliance partners and members of other groups [97, 98]. Chimpanzee males could be described as "psychopathic" due to high levels of sexual promiscuity and sexual coercion, impulsivity, and aggression, but they do not engage in parasitism. "Altruism" in chimpanzee society is reciprocal in nature and chimpanzees have exquisite memory for exchange partners and cheaters [97]. Chimpanzees do not provision one another with food as humans do [99]. Chimpanzee young are not fed by their mothers following weaning. Mothers allow young to feed beside them and to take food from them; however, they do not give food to their young. Juvenile chimpanzees assist their mothers by protecting and entertaining siblings; non-siblings do not practice allocare. Hence, the nature of chimpanzee society does not allow for the full expression of psychopathy.

Cooperative breeding in humans likely evolved out of a social structure similar to that of chimpanzees [92]. Attachment and competition thus shaped human society prior to the current social structure in which caregiving figures so prominently. Due to sexual conflict[5] the presence of allocare in females of a primate species tempers the dominance relations among males [100]. Recent evolution of the caregiving system may explain its absence in the percentage of the human population that is psychopathic. Anthropologists still do not agree as to when extended caregiving in humans evolved, but allocare may have begun with *Homo erectus* [101]. The invention of farming increased the rewards of parasitism (living off the labor of others). If psychopathy began with farming, it is a recently evolved human condition (10–15,000 years old).

10. Conclusions

The emotional and self-regulatory deficits of psychopathic personality have received much research attention with neglect of research into the motivational aspects of the disorder. The ethological framework provides a scaffold for a coherent motivational theory of psychopathy (**Table 1**). This theory proposes that the behaviors manifested by psychopathic individuals are caused by excessive and aberrant dominance responses and impaired salience attribution. The caregiving behavioral system and caring motivation is absent or highly disordered in psychopathic individuals. The sexual behavioral system of psychopathic individuals does not bond them with partners, and lack of bonding leads to sexual promiscuity and sexual coercion. Social ties are a "resource control strategy" for psychopathic individuals. Many maintain long-term social ties and show caregiving behaviors in the service of these ties which meet their material needs and power goals. It should be noted that without social ties, individuals who enjoy dominance, lack other individuals to dominate. Without willing helpers psychopathic persons could not survive or reproduce. Psychopathy is thus also a social disorder. Phylogenetic analysis reveals that chimpanzees (humans' closest extant related species) do not engage in caregiving; there are therefore there no parasitic chimpanzees. Chimpanzees are however, highly aggressive and do kill conspecifics, even alliance partners.

[5]Sexual conflict occurs when adaptation in one sex limit the expression of adaptations in the opposite sex.

Behavioral systems and motivation in psychopathy			
Behavioral system and associated goal	**Psychopathy and system internal working model**	**Psychopathy and system behaviors**	**Psychopathy and system social bonds**
Attachment system Goal: safety, security, physical needs met through others	Although psychopathic individuals are said not to "trust" others, family members and associates are viewed as sources of material sustenance and as sources of positive mirroring of self	Psychopathic individuals obtain material resources and positive self-mirroring from others through direct requests, conning and manipulation. Many adopt a parasitic lifestyle and are thus "dependent" on family members and associates	Attachment bonds serve the material and psychological needs of the psychopathic individual
Caregiving system Goal: to foster the well-being and growth of others	Psychopathic individuals appear to view themselves as the recipients of care from others. Their internal working models do not include the care of others. The common term for this internal working model is "sense of entitlement"	Deficits in emotional empathy prevent the assessment of and motivation to attend to the needs of others. Psychopathic individuals show profound deficits in caring behavior toward children, romantic partners, family members and associates	Caregiving bonds appear not to exist or to be very weak in psychopathic individuals
Sexual system Goal: mating and other sexual activities	Others are viewed as objects for sexual gratification	Precocious and promiscuous sexual activity may be central to psychopathy	Unrestricted sociosexuality with a failure to form sexual bonds with partners
Dominance system Goal: control over social and material resources	The presence of others activates the dominance system of psychopathic individuals. Others are viewed as objects to be controlled. Control by others is highly aversive to psychopathic individuals and is thus viewed negatively. Social hierarchies are salient	Interpersonal dominance through "prosocial" and coercive behaviors. Reciprocity and "charity" in the service of power goals. Psychopathic individuals seek attention and positive mirroring from others as feedback regarding superior status	Dominance bonds may exist. Psychopathic individuals behave as though they "own" others. They defend social connections with those they own to ensure physical and psychological needs are met

Table 1. Summary of human social behavioral systems as impacted by psychopathy.

Author details

Liane J. Leedom

Address all correspondence to: lleedom@bridgeport.edu

University of Bridgeport, Bridgeport, CT, USA

References

[1] Arnett PA. Autonomic responsivity in psychopaths: A critical review and theoretical proposal. Clinical Psychology Review. 1997 Dec;**17**(8):903-936

[2] Blair J, Mitchell D, Blair K. The Psychopath: Emotion and the Brain. Malden, MA: Blackwell; 2005. p. 212

[3] Hare RD, Neumann CS. Psychopathy. In: Oxford Textbook of Psychopathology. 2nd ed. [Internet]. New York, NY, US: Oxford University Press; 2009. pp. 622-650

[4] Partridge GE. Current conceptions of psychopathic personality. The American Journal of Psychiatry. 1930 Jul 1;**87**(1):53-99

[5] Nobel Media AB. The Nobel Prize in Physiology or Medicine 1973 [Internet]. NobelPrize.org. 2014 [cited 2017 Mar 12]. Available from: http://www.nobelprize.org/nobel_prizes/medicine/laureates/1973/

[6] Burkhardt RW. Patterns of Behavior: Konrad Lorenz, Niko Tinbergen, and the Founding of Ethology. Chicago, IL, US: University of Chicago Press; 2005. p. 649

[7] Baerends GP. Functional organization of behavior. In: Corner MA, Swaab DF, editors. Perspectives in Brain Research. New York, NY, US: Elsevier Biomedical Press; 2011. p. 427. (Progress in Brain Research; vol. 45)

[8] Tinbergen N. On aims and methods of ethology. Zeitschrift für Tierpsychologie. 1963; **20**(4):410-433

[9] Barlow, George W. Bateson, Peter P. G. (Ed); Klopfer, Peter H. (Ed). Has sociobiology killed ethology or revitalized it?. Perspectives in ethology, Vol. 8: Whither ethology?, (pp. 1-45). New York, NY, US: Plenum Press, xiv; 1989, 278 pp.

[10] Hinde RA, Grossmann KE, Grossmann K, Waters E. Ethology and attachment theory. In: Attachment for Infancy to Adulthood: The Major Longitudinal Studies. New York, NY, US: Guilford Press; 2005. pp. 1-12

[11] Leedom LJ. Human Social Behavioral Systems: Ethological framework for a unified theory. Human Ethology Bulletin. 2014;**29**:39-65

[12] Johnson SL, Leedom LJ, Muhtadie L. The dominance behavioral system and psychopathology: Evidence from self-report, observational, and biological studies. Psychological Bulletin. 2012 Apr 16;**138**(4):692-743

[13] Preston SD. The origins of altruism in offspring care. Psychological bulletin. 2013;**139.6**: 1305-1321

[14] Bowlby J. (1944). Forty-four juvenile thieves: Their characters and home life. International Journal of Psycho-Analysis, 25, 19-52

[15] Bowlby J. Attachment and Loss: Volume 2. Separation. New York, NY, US: Basic Books; 1973

[16] Bowlby J. By ethology out of psycho-analysis: An experiment in interbreeding. Animal Behaviour. 1980;**28**(3):649-656

[17] Flagel SB, Akil H, Robinson TE. Individual differences in the attribution of incentive salience to reward-related cues: Implications for addiction. Neuropharmacology. 2009;**56**(Suppl 1):139-148

[18] Goldstein RZ, Volkow ND. Drug addiction and its underlying neurobiological basis: Neuroimaging evidence for the involvement of the frontal cortex. The American Journal of Psychiatry. 2002 Oct 1;**159**(10):1642-1652

[19] Depue RA, Morrone-Strupinsky JV. A neurobehavioral model of affiliative bonding: Implications for conceptualizing a human trait of affiliation. Behavioral and Brain Sciences. 2005 Jun;**28**(3):313-395

[20] Feldman R, Weller A, Zagoory-Sharon O, Levine A. Evidence for a neuroendocrinological foundation of human affiliation: Plasma oxytocin levels across pregnancy and the postpartum period predict mother-infant bonding. Psychological Science. 2007;**18**(11):965-970

[21] Fuentes A. Patterns and trends in primate pair bonds. International Journal of Primatology. 2002 Oct;**23**(5):953-978

[22] Shaver PR, Mikulincer M. A behavioral systems approach to romantic love relationships: Attachment, caregiving, and sex. In: Sternberg RJ, Weis K, editors. The New Psychology of Love. New Haven, CT, US: Yale University Press; 2006. pp. 35-64

[23] Maslow AH. A theory of human motivation. Psychological Review. 1943 Jul;**50**(4): 370-396

[24] Kernberg OF. Pathological narcissism and narcissistic personality disorder: Theoretical background and diagnostic classification. In: Ronningstam EF, editor. Disorders of Narcissism: Diagnostic, Clinical, and Empirical Implications. Washington, DC, US: American Psychiatric Association; 1998. pp. 29-51

[25] McCord W, McCord J. Psychopathy and Delinquency. [Internet]. Oxford, England: Grune and Stratton; 1956

[26] Brody Y, Rosenfeld B. Object relations in criminal psychopaths. International Journal of Offender Therapy and Comparative Criminology. 2002 Aug;**46**(4):400-411

[27] American Psychiatric Association DSM-5 Personality Disorders Work Group. Proposed Revision | APA DSM-5 [Internet]. 2010 [cited 2010 Feb 10]. Available from: http://www.dsm5.org/ProposedRevisions/Pages/proposedrevision.aspx?rid=16#

[28] Cleckley HM. The Mask of Sanity: An Attempt to Clarify Some Issues about the So-called Psychopathic Personality. St. Louis, MO: C. V. Mosby Co.; 1964. p. 520

[29] Fersch E. Thinking About Psychopaths and Psychopathy: Answers to Frequently Asked Questions With Case Examples. iUniverse, Inc.; Lincoln, NE USA. 2006

[30] Leedom LJ, Bass A, Almas LH. The problem of parental psychopathy. Journal of Child Custody. 2013;**10**(2):154-184

[31] Leedom LJ, Geislin E, Hartoonian Almas L. "Did he ever love me?" A qualitative study of life with a psychopathic husband. Family & Intimate Partner Violence Quarterly. 2013;**5**(2):103-135

[32] Morehead P. Green River Serial Killer—Biography of an Unsuspecting Wife. 1st ed. Wellesley, MA: Branden Books; 2007

[33] Gawda B. Syntax of emotional narratives of persons diagnosed with antisocial personality. Journal of Psycholinguistic Research. 2010;**39**(4):273-283

[34] Leedom LJ, Andersen D. Antisocial/psychopathic personality: What do family members, romantic partners and friends report? Society for the Scientific Study of Psychopathy Montreal, Canada; 2011

[35] Dutton DG, Golant SK. The Batterer: A Psychological Profile. New York, NY, US: Basic Books; 1997. p. 230

[36] Lynam DR, Widiger TA. Using a general model of personality to identify the basic elements of psychopathy. Journal of Personality Disorders. 2007 Apr;**21**(2):160-178

[37] Skeem J, Johansson P, Andershed H, Kerr M, Louden JE. Two subtypes of psychopathic violent offenders that parallel primary and secondary variants. Journal of Abnormal Psychology. 2007 May;**116**(2):395-409

[38] Cale EM, Lilienfeld SO. Psychopathy factors and risk for aggressive behavior: A test of the "threatened egotism" hypothesis. Law and Human Behavior. 2006 Feb;**30**(1):51-74

[39] Picardi A, Caroppo E, Toni A, Bitetti D, Di Maria G. Stability of attachment-related anxiety and avoidance and their relationships with the five-factor model and the psychobiological model of personality. Psychology and Psychotherapy: Theory, Research and Practice. 2005;**78**(3):327-345

[40] Ali F, Chamorro-Premuzic T. The dark side of love and life satisfaction: Associations with intimate relationships, psychopathy and Machiavellianism. Personality and Individual Differences. 2010 Jan;**48**(2):228-233

[41] Savard C, Sabourin S, Lussier Y. Male sub-threshold psychopathic traits and couple distress. Personality and Individual Differences. 2006 Apr;**40**(5):931-942

[42] Russell LA. Examination of the Psychopathic Personality Inventory-revised and the Psychopathy Construct in a College Sample. [Internet]. [US]: ProQuest Information & Learning; 2005

[43] Dillinger RJ. An Exploration of the Interpersonal Features of Psychopathy. [Internet]. [US]: ProQuest Information & Learning; 2008

[44] Brennan KA, Shaver PR. Attachment styles and personality disorders: Their connections to each other and to parental divorce, parental death, and perceptions of parental caregiving. Journal of Personality. 1998 Oct;**66**(5):835-878

[45] Ross T, Pfäfflin F. Attachment and interpersonal problems in a prison environment. Journal of Forensic Psychiatry & Psychology. 2007 Mar;**18**(1):90-98

[46] Frodi A, Dernevik M, Sepa A, Philipson J, Bragesjö M. Current attachment representations of incarcerated offenders varying in degree of psychopathy. Attachment & Human Development. 2001 Dec;**3**(3):269-283

[47] van IJzendoorn MH, Feldbrugge JTTM, Derks FCH, de Ruiter C, Verhagen MFM, Philipse MWG, et al. Attachment representations of personality-disordered criminal offenders. American Journal of Orthopsychiatry. 1997 Jul;**67**(3):449-459

[48] Rosenstein DS, Horowitz HA. Attachment, personality, and psychopathology: Relationship as a regulatory context in adolescence. Adolescent Psychiatry. 1993;**19**:150-176

[49] Blackburn R, Maybury C. Identifying the psychopath: The relation of Cleckley's criteria to the interpersonal domain. Personality and Individual Differences. 1985;**6**(3):375-386

[50] Colwell JT. An interpersonal method for scoring the tat: Implications for distinguishing individuals with psychopathic symptomatology using Leary's circumplex model. [doctoral dissertation]. [US]: Rosalind Franklin University; 1998

[51] Decety J, Skelly LR, Kiehl KA. Brain response to empathy-eliciting scenarios involving pain in incarcerated individuals with psychopathy. JAMA Psychiatry. 2013 Jun 1;**70**(6):638

[52] American Psychiatric Association. Diagnostic and Statistical Manual of Mental Disorders. 3rd ed., text rev. American Psychiatric Association Press; Washington, DC, US; 1987

[53] Bosquet M, Egeland B. Predicting parenting behaviors from Antisocial Practices content scale scores of the MMPI-2 administered during pregnancy. Journal of Personality Assessment. 2000 Feb;**74**(1):146-162

[54] Taylor MC. Psychopathy and Attachment in a Group of Incarcerated Females. [Internet]. [US]: ProQuest Information & Learning; 1998

[55] Kirkman CA. From soap opera to science: Towards gaining access to the psychopaths who live amongst us. Psychology and Psychotherapy. 2005 Sep;**78**(Pt 3):379-396

[56] Marshall AD, Holtzworth-Munroe A. Recognition of wives' emotional expressions: A mechanism in the relationship between psychopathology and intimate partner violence perpetration. Journal of Family Psychology. 2010 Feb;**24**(1):21-30

[57] Decety J, Michalska KJ, Akitsuki Y, Lahey BB. Atypical empathic responses in adolescents with aggressive conduct disorder: A functional MRI investigation. Biological Psychology. 2009 Feb;**80**(2):203-211

[58] Gillstrom BJ, Hare RD. Language-related hand gestures in psychopaths. Journal of Personality Disorders. 1988;**2**(1):21-27

[59] Rimé B, Bouvy H, Leborgne B, Rouillon F. Psychopathy and nonverbal behavior in an interpersonal situation. Journal of Abnormal Psychology. 1978 Dec;**87**(6):636-643

[60] Bursten B. The manipulative personality. Archives of General Psychiatry. 1972 Apr;**26**(4): 318-321

[61] Widom CS, Katkin FS, Stewart AJ, Fondacaro M. Multivariate analysis of personality and motivation in female delinquents. Journal of Research in Crime and Delinquency. 1983 Jul;**20**(2):277-290

[62] Endres J. The language of the psychopath: Characteristics of prisoners' performance in a sentence completion test. Criminal Behaviour and Mental Health. 2004;**14**(3):214-226

[63] Klein A. Grand Deception the World's Most Spectacular and Successful Haxes, Impostures, Ruses and Frauds. New York, NY, US: J B Lippincott Co; 1955

[64] Hoff HA, Rypdal K, Hystad SW, Hart SD, Mykletun A, Kreis MKF, et al. Cross-language consistency of the Comprehensive Assessment of Psychopathic Personality (CAPP) model. Personality Disorders: Theory, Research, and Treatment. 2014 Oct;**5**(4):356-368

[65] Hoff HA, Rypdal K, Mykletun A, Cooke DJ. A prototypicality validation of the Comprehensive Assessment of Psychopathic Personality (CAPP). Journal of Personality Disorders. 2012 Jun;**26**(3):414-427

[66] Smith ST, Edens JF, Clark J, Rulseh A. "So, what is a psychopath?" Venireperson perceptions, beliefs, and attitudes about psychopathic personality. Law and Human Behavior. 2014 Oct;**38**(5):490-500

[67] Sörman K, Edens JF, Smith ST, Svensson O, Howner K, Kristiansson M, et al. Forensic mental health professionals' perceptions of psychopathy: A prototypicality analysis of the Comprehensive Assessment of Psychopathic Personality in Sweden. Law and Human Behavior. 2014 Oct;**38**(5):405-417

[68] Kosson DS, Steuerwald BL, Forth AE, Kirkhart KJ. A new method for assessing the interpersonal behavior of psychopathic individuals: Preliminary validation studies. Psychological Assessment. 1997 Jun;**9**(2):89-101

[69] Schenley A. Correlational Analysis of Psychopathic Personality Traits in Male and Female Offenders: A Multitrait-multimethod Approach. [US]: ProQuest Information & Learning; 2003

[70] Zolondek S, Lilienfeld SO, Patrick CJ, Fowler KA. The interpersonal measure of psychopathy: Construct and incremental validity in male prisoners. Assessment. 2006 Dec;**13**(4):470-482

[71] Salekin RT, Trobst KK, Krioukova M. Construct validity of psychopathy in a community sample: A nomological net approach. Journal of Personality Disorders. 2001 Oct;**15**(5):425-441

[72] Reidy DE, Wilson LF, Sloan CA, Cohn AM, Smart LM, Zeichner A. Psychopathic traits and men's anger response to interpersonal conflict: A pilot study. Personality and Individual Differences. 2013 Nov;**55**(8):957-961

[73] Reidy DE, Zeichner A, Martinez MA. Effects of psychopathy traits on unprovoked aggression. Aggressive Behavior. 2008 Jun 5;**34**(3):319-328

[74] Seibert LA, Miller JD, Few LR, Zeichner A, Lynam DR. An examination of the structure of self-report psychopathy measures and their relations with general traits and externalizing behaviors. Personality Disorders: Theory, Research, and Treatment. 2011 Jul;**2**(3):193-208

[75] Reidy DE, Shelley-Tremblay JF, Lilienfeld SO. Psychopathy, reactive aggression, and precarious proclamations: A review of behavioral, cognitive, and biological research. Aggression and Violent Behavior. 2011 Nov;**16**(6):512-524

[76] Goncalves MK, Campbell L. The Dark Triad and the derogation of mating competitors. Personality and Individual Differences. 2014 Sep;**67**:42-46

[77] Schmitt DP, Shackelford TK. Big Five traits related to short-term mating: From personality to promiscuity across 46 nations. Evolutionary Psychology. 2008;**6**(2):246-282

[78] Linton DK, Wiener NI. Personality and potential conceptions: Mating success in a modern Western male sample. Personality and Individual Differences. 2001 Oct;**31**(5): 675-688

[79] Wilson D, Manual A, Lavelle S. Personality characteristics of Zimbabwean men who visit prostitutes: Implications for AIDS prevention programmes. Personality and Individual Differences. 1992 Mar;**13**(3):275-279

[80] Zuckerman M. The neurobiology of impulsive sensation seeking: Genetics, brain physiology, biochemistry, and neurology. In: Neurobiology of Exceptionality [Internet]. New York, NY, US: Kluwer Academic/Plenum Publishers; 2005. pp. 31-52. Available from: http://search.ebscohost.com/login.aspx?direct=true&db=psyh&AN=2005-04213-002&site=ehost-live

[81] Zuckerman M, Kuhlman DM, Joireman J, Teta P, Kraft M. A comparison of three structural models for personality: The Big Three, the Big Five, and the Alternative Five. Journal of Personality and Social Psychology. 1993 Oct;**65**(4):757-768

[82] Barta WD, Kiene SM. Motivations for infidelity in heterosexual dating couples: The roles of gender, personality differences, and sociosexual orientation. Journal of Social and Personal Relationships. 2005 Jun;**22**(3):339-360

[83] Jonason PK, Kavanagh P. The dark side of love: Love styles and the Dark Triad. Personality and Individual Differences. 2010 Oct;**49**(6):606-610

[84] Miller JD, Jones SE, Lynam DR. Psychopathic traits from the perspective of self and informant reports: Is there evidence for a lack of insight? Journal of Abnormal Psychology. 2011 Aug;**120**(3):758-764

[85] Outcalt J. The Romantic Relationships Associated with Psychopathy: Approach or Avoidance? [Internet]. [US]: ProQuest Information & Learning; 2008

[86] Harris GT, Rice ME, Hilton NZ, Lalumière ML, Quinsey VL. Coercive and precocious sexuality as a fundamental aspect of psychopathy. Journal of Personality Disorders. 2007 Feb;**21**(1):1-27

[87] Shiota MN, Keltner D, John OP. Positive emotion dispositions differentially associated with Big Five personality and attachment style. The Journal of Positive Psychology. 2006 Apr;**1**(2):61-71

[88] van den Bos W, Golka PJM, Effelsberg D, McClure SM. Pyrrhic victories: The need for social status drives costly competitive behavior. Frontiers in Neuroscience [Internet]. 2013 Oct 23 [cited 2014 Dec 20];**7**:1-11. Available from: http://www.ncbi.nlm.nih.gov/pmc/articles/PMC3805938/

[89] Harlow HF. Learning to Love. Oxford, England: Ballantine; 1973

[90] Coyne SM, Thomas TJ. Psychopathy, aggression, and cheating behavior: A test of the Cheater-Hawk hypothesis. Personality and Individual Differences. 2008 Apr;**44**(5):1105-1115

[91] Mealey L. The sociobiology of sociopathy: An integrated evolutionary model. Behavioral and Brain Sciences. 1995;**18**(3):523-599

[92] Van Schaik CP, Burkart J. Mind the gap: Cooperative breeding and the evolution of our unique features. In: Mind the Gap: Tracing the Origins of Human Universals. New York, NY, US: Springer; 2010. pp. 477-497

[93] Buss DM, Haselton MG, Shackelford TK, Bleske AL, Wakefield JC. Adaptations, exaptations, and spandrels. American Psychologist. 1998;**53**(5):533-548

[94] Leedom LJ. Is psychopathy a disorder or an adaptation?. Frontiers in Evolutionary Psychology. 2012;**549**:549-550

[95] Archer J. Testosterone and human aggression: An evaluation of the challenge hypothesis. Neuroscience & Biobehavioral Reviews. 2006;**30**(3):319-345

[96] Goodall J. Infant killing and cannibalism in free-living chimpanzees. Folia Primatologica. 1977;**28**(4):259-289

[97] de Waal FB. Chimpanzee Politics: Power and Sex Among the Apes. Revised Edition. Baltimore, MD, USA: The John Hopkins University Press; 1998. p. 235

[98] Watts DP, Muller M, Amsler SJ, Mbabazi G, Mitani JC. Lethal intergroup aggression by chimpanzees in Kibale National Park, Uganda. American Journal of Primatology. 2006 Feb;**68**(2):161-180

[99] Jaeggi AV, Stevens JMG, Van Schaik CP. Tolerant food sharing and reciprocity is precluded by despotism among bonobos but not chimpanzees. American Journal of Physical Anthropology. 2010 Sep;**143**(1):41-51

[100] Thierry B, Iwaniuk AN, Pellis SM. The influence of phylogeny on the social behaviour of macaques (Primates: Cercopithecidae, genus *Macaca*). Ethology. 2000 Aug 1;**106**(8):713-728

[101] O'connell JF, Hawkes K, Blurton Jones NG. Grandmothering and the evolution of *Homo erectus*. Journal of Human Evolution. 1999 May;**36**(5):461-485

Chapter 7

The Impact of Psychopathy on the Family

Liane J. Leedom

Additional information is available at the end of the chapter

http://dx.doi.org/10.5772/intechopen.70227

Abstract

Psychopathy is the amalgamation of personality disorder traits associated with criminal and other antisocial behavior. Although current theory postulates that psychopathic individuals do not form lasting bonds with others, this chapter provides ample evidence that psychopathic individuals are highly social and maintain ties over years. Psychopathic individuals have relationships with friends, co-workers, relatives, siblings, parents, romantic partners, and children. These relationships serve their social and material needs. This chapter presents all available studies to date on the friendship, filial, sibling, partnering, and parenting behavior of psychopathic individuals. The impact of psychopathic individuals on organizational and family functioning is also addressed.

Keywords: antisocial personality disorder, psychopathy, coercive control, intimate partner violence, child abuse, intergenerational transmission, parenting

1. Introduction: psychopathy a family problem

The belief that psychopathic individuals do not form lasting bonds with others [1], arguments over nomenclature[1] and lack of research outside of forensic settings have hindered study of psychopathy and the family. Although the connection between psychopathy and crime perpetration is well-documented, rate of victimization of friends and relatives is unknown [2, 3]. Intrafamilial physical, sexual, psychological, and financial abuse is the subject of epidemiologic investigations; however, the connection between familial victimization

[1]The term psychopathy is used in this chapter to refer to a disorder that is dimensional. This chapter does not distinguish between ASPD, psychopathy and pathological narcissism beyond discussing the differential impact of PCL-R Factors 1 and 2 symptoms on family members and friends. Lay people most often use the terms "sociopath" or "narcissist" to refer to a person with psychopathy. So-called "narcissists" described by lay people victimize others and manifest the interpersonal behaviors and affective deficits of psychopathy; they may lack a criminal record and closely correspond to the "successful psychopaths" described in the research literature.

and symptoms of psychopathy in perpetrators is not established. If psychopathy is indeed the *Unified Theory of Crime* [4], risk for family and friend victimization likely increases linearly or perhaps exponentially with symptoms of the disorder. Two recent handbooks regarding psychopathy and law have chapters outlining family psychopathy and its legal consequences, but little data are presented in them [5, 6]. None of the most authoritative edited academic books regarding psychopathy published between 2001 and 2015 contains any discussion on the impact of psychopathic individuals on their family members and friends [7–11]. In this chapter, case vignettes and a comprehensive overview of available quantitative and qualitative studies are presented to motivate and provide a framework for further investigation.

Cleckley mentioned the plight of numerous family members in 15 case studies he presented in *The Mask of Sanity* (**Table 1**) [12]. Although Cleckley's writing is over 60 years old, descriptions of psychopathic individuals' relationships have not changed. One recent edited book [13] details the initial evaluation of "Frank" an individual with psychopathic traits. Like Cleckley, the evaluating clinician obtained history from family members when Frank himself was not forthcoming with information. The psychosocial history described Frank's victimization of family members including his younger brother, maternal aunt, maternal grandparents, two cousins, pets, lifelong friend, and wife. Frank's case illustrates the extent to which community clinicians rely on family members when evaluating and treating individuals with psychopathy [14]. The impact of psychopathic individuals on family members is thus well known to clinicians who have heard numerous detailed accounts of victimization during history taking. Clinicians are also aware of psychopathy when there is a co-occurring substance use disorder. Co-occurring substance use disorders, gambling, and "sex addiction" place additional stress on the family, above and beyond that caused by psychopathy.

The plight of family members of psychopathic individuals (a predominant theme in 14/15 cases reported in Cleckley's *Mask of Sanity*)

Family relationship	Hardship endured
Parents	Regarding "Walter's" father, "His grief and shame seemed almost, but not quite too much for him"
	Regarding "Roberta," "such conduct of course suggests she might have been deliberately trying to hurt her parents"
	"Stanley's" mother is quoted, "...and it's just killing us, all the things he does"
Siblings	"Jack's" story, "In time he became an all but unbearable burden on the other members of his family (4 siblings)"
Spouses	Spouses are described in 9 cases, suffering desertion, financial abuse, infidelity and assault (2 cases)
Children	Children are only mentioned in two cases and no details are given regarding parenting behavior

Table 1. Family members in 14/15 cases detailed in Cleckley's *Mask of Sanity*.

Although epidemiologic data are lacking, it is possible to estimate the scope of the problem of family psychopathy using data from "Frank" and the United States Census as a model. The prevalence of antisocial personality disorder (ASPD) is about 4% of the adult population [15] and severe psychopathy may be 0.06% [16]; there are 219,726,708 adults between 18 and 65 years in the USA [17]. Hence, there are an estimated 8.8 million individuals with ASPD including 1.3 million with severe psychopathy. If Frank is typical of those with moderate psychopathy and each person with ASPD adversely affects eight close others, then the public health problem of psychopathy may impact 70.4 million Americans or nearly a third of the adult population. Given the familial nature of personality and related disorders, many impacted individuals also have their own psychiatric morbidity, and many families are coping with more than one psychopathic individual [18].

2. Psychopathic sons/daughters: coercion starts early

To coerce means to compel or force another to comply. Coercive behavior reflects reactance and a motive to dominate others; it is a tool for obtaining control over resources and other people [19, 20]. Patterson identified "coercive family interactions" that occur in the families of children and teens with the externalizing disorders that are precursors to adult psychopathy. He hypothesized that children learn coercion tactics early in life because such tactics are an effective strategy for the procurement of reinforcers. Strong dominance motivation facilitates learning of coercive tactics because dominant individuals are sensitive to reward [19]. Coercion is associated with negative emotions—trait anger and irritability (these often accompany trait dominance motivation [19]). According to Patterson, "It is the patterned irritable exchanges between the problem child, his mother, and his siblings that define the 'basic training' for coercion" [21]. Patterson brilliantly observed that not only is the problem child trained in coercion during these family interactions, but also parents are trained to submit to the child who uses coercive tactics: the externalizing child asks for something; parent refuses, child then escalates his/her demands until the parent submits. The difference between normative and problem children is that the former are not excessively driven to dominate their parents and problem children are not hampered in their demands by the presence of empathy [22]. Because problem children are deficient in (or dissociate from) emotional empathy, they are not concerned that their behavior distresses their parents.

Children's coercive behavior and lack of rewarding child-parent interaction has negative effects on parents' attributions and behavior [23]. Parents of problem children are more likely to view the motives of their children as malevolent. Negative parenting behavior results from the impact of the child's externalizing disorder on the parent; it is not necessarily the sole cause of the problem child's behavior. Because problem children emotionally drain their parents, they are robbed of the opportunity to learn enjoyment of affection and empathy in their relationships with them. Studies of the causes of psychopathy reveal that genes contribute about half of the risk; the rest of the risk primarily comes from a child's unique environment [24]. Therefore, the dysfunctional relationships between problem children and their parents are likely to be important to developmental continuity of disorder. Treatment of externalizing children involves helping parents break the cycle of coercion and negativity, and cultivate affectionate interactions [25, 26].

While some parents of children with externalizing disorders also have psychopathic traits, many do not. These unaffected parents suffer a great deal trying to meet the needs of their disordered children who age to maturity but often are not independent (**Table 1**). Parents continue to give care and may be subjected to parasitism and abuse [12, 14]. In my work, I have interviewed many mothers and fathers who partnered and had children with psychopathic men and women. I discovered that when the children from these relationships develop psychopathy, it becomes impossible for these parents to escape the victimization experience that began with their psychopathic partner. In middle adulthood, they find that the life-energy expended parenting was spent on a child who now preys on others and is unable to assume adult roles. The golden years many dreamt of living, with grandchildren and mature relationships with adult sons and daughters are fraught with loneliness and stress.

3. Psychopathic siblings

Most children in Western countries have at least one sibling, therefore most psychopathic individuals have a sibling [27, 28]. Sibling abuse is the most common form of domestic abuse [29], and sibling sexual abuse is the most common form of familial sexual abuse [30]. Sibling violence reflects risk for violent behavior generally and hence may point to psychopathic traits [31]. Sibling assault leading to injury is linked to psychopathy [31]. Despite these statistics, the impact of children with externalizing disorders on their siblings and the extent to which sibling abuse is associated with morbidity in either perpetrators or victims is not well documented. Patterson [32], and his group described two ways older siblings increase risk for antisocial behavior in younger siblings. First, externalizing children train their siblings in coercion. This training results from both imitation of coercive interactions with parents and from direct practice in coercive behavior during sibling conflict. Second, externalizing siblings recruit their younger brothers and sisters into antisocial activities **(Table 2**) [33].

One study directly examined dyadic interactions between antisocial teens and a same sex sibling, friend, and romantic partner during problem-solving tasks. Negative dyadic interactions included: (a) negative verbal statements (e.g., disapproval) and (b) nonverbal behavior (e.g., negative facial expressions); (c) verbal attacks (e.g., name calling); (d) coercive and ambiguous coercive behavior (e.g., threatening directives that express a demand); (e) requests and ambiguous requests; (f) commands and ambiguous commands (e.g., directives); and (g) physical aggression (e.g., shoving) [34]. These interactions occurred at a relatively high rate, and interestingly, although the teens treated siblings and romantic partners coercively, they were less aggressive toward their friends. The researchers observed a high rate of talking about antisocial activities with siblings. Antisocial talk predicted persistence of antisocial behavior into adulthood. Such verbal exchanges reflect the assumption of an antisocial identity that may be imparted to younger siblings. Dominance relations in adolescent romantic relationships resemble familial relationships more than they do friendships—evidence that schemas of coercion learned in early family interactions are directly transferred to schemas regarding sexual partnerships (see Section 5).

http://dx.doi.org/10.5772/intechopen.70227

My stepfather sexually molested me when I was eight. My sister who was nine, was also molested; I know because I saw him go to her. We never talked about what happened. When she was 20, I asked her and she denied it then admitted it happened to her when I said I saw him. My father was shot and killed when we were very young. He used drugs and had a bad temper, so someone shot him. My sister was always wild when we were growing up. We fought a lot and there wasn't much affection in my family.
My sister has been sexually promiscuous since her teen years. I never had any friends because if she would find out that I had a friend, she would have sex with that friend's boyfriend. My mother would say I had to stick up for my sister. But, my sister has sex with nearly every man she knows. When she sees a married couple, she wants what they have, so she sleeps with the husband. When he leaves his wife to be with her, she grows tired and drops him. My sister has been with all kinds of men, black, white and Hispanic. She becomes whatever that man is. When she's with a black, she acts black. She's white when she's with a white guy.
I don't think my sister ever uses protection when she has sex, look she had a baby a year ago. I don't know how she can do this to herself...all those men. According to a friend of mine, the men in the town even talk about my sister. They have all had sex with her and think she's good. I left home when I was 16 because my sister convinced me that my mother didn't want me. She often told me that my mother didn't like me. My sister told me a lot of things my mother didn't really say. My sister has two children that I worry about, especially her son who is seven. She switches men every few months, each time there is a new guy she says to her son, "This is your father." Then when she gets tired of the guy, she gets rid of him and her son never sees the man again. She left her son's father when he was in jail. Her son's father has 8 kids and he only cares for two of them. My nephew has problems and my sister just ignores him. She is into her baby now. The baby girl is one. I don't think she knows who the baby's father is. My sister spends all her money on the men in her life, while her children go without clothes and doctor visits. She never pays any of her bills. She has furniture from a rental place she never paid then moved away with the furniture. She doesn't feel she should have to pay any of her bills. She has a job. She keeps it because she lies to her boss and makes her feel sorry for her. She tells everyone that she is a single mother and that she has no family. She is a single mother, but we want to help her. My sister is not sorry for any of the bad things she has done. Instead, she lies to cover things up. It seems she believes her own lies. I can't believe how much my sister lies. She doesn't tell the truth about anything.
My sister is beautiful and very nice. I keep thinking she is a good person, then when I think about the way she treats my nephew, I get mad. She says she doesn't want him, but she won't give him to us. She wants to be in control. I keep thinking that my sister acts this way because she was molested. My mother says she has always been wild and difficult. Even when my father was alive, she was oppositional. I remember she did everything he told her not to do. Although my sister does not steal from my mother, she takes advantage of her. If my mother has a boyfriend, my sister will call him behind my mother's back, and ask him for favors, even if he and my mom aren't that close. Although my sister doesn't admit to having any problems, she blames my mother for everything. My mother never showed us any affection.

Table 2. "Mary" describes life with her sister. This written account was provided by a woman who wanted her story shared to help others. The account is hers and illustrates the familial nature of psychopathy and the plight of those exposed to psychopathy in multiple family members; details were altered to further conceal "Mary's" identity.

4. Psychopathic friends

> *"An insincere and evil friend is more to be feared than a wild beast; a wild beast may wound your body, but an evil friend will wound your mind."*—Buddha

In this discussion, the terms "friend" and "companion" are synonymous such that a friend is a preferred, familiar companion. In my role as professor of psychology and psychopathy researcher, I have been approached by members of the public, students, and staff who have shared their stories of friendship with psychopathic individuals. I am impressed by the level of lasting distress caused by abuse from psychopathic friends. It is not unexpected that psychopathic individuals maintain familial ties that serve their material needs; it is contrary to current theory that many also actively cultivate friendships. Current theory should be amended to account for sociability in psychopathic individuals. Studies by Kosson demonstrate that psychopathy is negatively associated with schizoid personality or a preference for solitary activities [35]. That psychopathic individuals report companions is further evidence for the idea that they do not prefer to be alone. Although psychopathic individuals may lack "affection," there is some reward connected to the company of others. If psychopathy produced an indifference to companionship, theory would predict that psychopathic individuals would be loners and that they would be less likely than other offenders to join gangs. The social nature of psychopathy is evidenced by the positive association between gang membership and psychopathy and between gang leadership and the interpersonal features of psychopathy [36, 37]. The interpersonal features of psychopathy are also positively associated with social bonds in prison [38]. If psychopathic individuals are truly devoid of affection, these observations challenge the notion that affection and caring are necessary determinants of human social ties.

4.1. What motivates psychopathic individuals to cultivate friendships?

There are three sources of information regarding psychopathy and friendship: forensic studies, surveys of the general population, and anecdotal accounts. Forensic studies support the social nature of psychopathy indicating that it is associated with co-offending as opposed to solo-offending [39]. Accordingly, psychopathy does not reduce the likelihood of gang membership and gang membership appears to causally relate to callous-unemotional traits [36, 37]. Forensic studies demonstrate the interactive nature of friendship and personality traits. Psychopathy may predispose to the choice of antisocial friends and gang membership and in turn, these associations strengthen the stability of psychopathic personality traits [36]. In college students, DSM 5, Section 111 personality traits associated with ASPD including antagonism, correlate with attempts to be close to others and warm as opposed to cold dominant behavior (as reported by friends) [40]. There is also no negative association between psychopathy and the need to belong in young adults [41]. Community studies of psychopathy in adolescents demonstrate that youth high in psychopathic traits are "as likely as others to have important peers in their lives," though these friendships may have less temporal stability [42]. Adolescents tend to associate with friends who have similar levels of psychopathy and friends engage in antisocial behavior (including substance abuse) together [39]. Psychopathy is associated with more reciprocated relationships in male adolescents, and does not affect levels of perceived support in relationships. As with adolescents, adults associate with others who have similar levels of psychopathy [43]. In contrast to forensic settings, psychopathy in college settings may not be associated with leadership [44]. Psychopathy is moderately associated with self-reports of not helping friends [31].

In summary, although psychopathy may cause friendships to have less temporal stability, psychopathic individuals seek out companionship and engage in their preferred activities with others. Researchers have labeled such relationships "shallow" and "lacking in depth" because psychopathy is associated with low closeness and reduced helping [31]. That psychopathic individuals cultivate friends to meet their material and companionship needs, receive admiration and attention, and to dominate others is supported by anecdotal accounts [2, 45]. Clinicians and researchers should work to better understand the nature of social reinforcement for psychopathic individuals. Informed application (or deprivation) of social reinforcement has the potential to enhance individual, group, and family therapy for psychopathic adolescents and adults.

4.2. How are friends and friendship affected by psychopathy?

> *"Friendship does not mean the same thing to them. They'll use the word love a lot, but they really don't know what love means. They've never properly experienced it"* [46]—Adrian Raine, Ph. D.

Individuals with psychopathy seek relationships to meet material and companionship needs. They then abuse and often fail to help others. This dynamic creates difficulties for friends with low levels of psychopathic traits (who have different relationship expectations). I find that such friends are distressed and perplexed by abuse, betrayals, and lack of reciprocity (also noted in [6]). Friends are often very reluctant to sever ties with psychopathic individuals even those who have abused them. This reluctance reflects both effective manipulation on the part of the psychopathic friend and the presence of a social bond. I could not find any research regarding whether psychopathic individuals leave relationships on their own accord or whether relationships are terminated by abused friends. There is also no systematic data available regarding the time and energy psychopathic individuals invest in maintaining their friendships. Anecdotal data from spouses verify that even highly psychopathic individuals do invest energy into friendships [47].

4.3. How is a social network affected by the level of psychopathy in its individual members?

Psychopathic individuals impact their friendship networks in addition to impacting individual friends. There is too little information regarding psychopathic traits and gangs to make definitive statements about the way individual psychopathy impacts the organization of the gang collective. Decker and Curry state that members murder their "brothers" and that gang murders are often related to intra- as opposed to intergang rivalry. They also suggest that gangs are not well organized [48]. Murder of associates and lack of organization could result from psychopathy in gang members. Poor organization could result from the impaired executive function in members related to the lifestyle facet of psychopathy [49]. Non-criminal organizations are also impacted by members' psychopathy. In corporations, psychopathy is associated with passive leadership [50] and employee dissatisfaction with supervision [51]. Anecdotal evidence suggests that psychopathy is related to corporate crime and organizational dysfunction [52]. The impact of psychopathy on family organization is discussed below. In the family, facets of PCL-R psychopathy have differential effects on functional dynamics.

5. Psychopathy and romantic partnerships

Sexual promiscuity and multiple short-term marital relationships are part of the definition of psychopathy [53, 54]. Psychopathy is associated with a ludic love style and self-reports of uncommitted sex (**Table 3**) [55]. These symptoms convey the impression that psychopathic individuals easily navigate from one relationship to the next without much investment. Lack of investment and ease of relationship mobility would be consistent with the view that psychopathy is associated with a lack of social bonds. Unfortunately for victims and theories

Studies of Psychopathy and Romantic Relationships			
N	**Definition of psychopathic traits**	**Study Findings**	**Study Publication year [Reference]**
431 (Individuals)	LSRP	Psychopathy associated with low well-being and ill-being. Psychopathy associated with relationship quality measures. Relationship quality measures mediated link between psychopathy and well (ill)-being. Effects stronger for women	2010 [18]
297 (Individuals)	LSRP	Primary psychopathy was positively associated with latent relationship factor. Secondary psychopathy was negatively associated with life satisfaction and intimacy. Psychopathy and sociosexual orientation equally related to commitment	2016 [59]
45 (Couples)	SRP-II	Psychopathy associated with assortative mating and decreased relationship satisfaction in dating couples	2014 [68]
140 (Couples)	LSRP	In men, primary and secondary psychopathy associated with own attachment anxiety and avoidance and partner's attachment anxiety and attachment avoidance Psychopathic traits in women correlated with own and partner's attachment anxiety and avoidance. Assortative mating was for primary psychopathic traits	2015 [69]
140 (Couples)	LSRP	Neuroticism linked to global, primary and secondary psychopathy. Perpetration of psychological aggression linked to global, primary and secondary psychopathy Relationship satisfaction negatively related to secondary psychopathy Assortative mating: primary > global > secondary psychopathic traits	2011 [70]
152 (Couples)	LSRP	Dyadic adjustment related to global and secondary psychopathy in men. Relationship distress at Time 1 associated with increases in men's psychopathy scores a year later (Time 2)	2006 [71]
1805 (Couples)	DSM III-R	Adult antisocial behavior and CD linked to negative dyadic adjustment; effect not fully explained by low constraint	2010 [72]
1255 (Couples)	DSM III-R	Adult antisocial behavior associated with lower cohesion, satisfaction, consensus on important issues and affective expression	2013 [73]
1408 (Couples)	DSM III-R	Assortative mating for CD. History of CD linked to marital discord and decreased family adaptability	2000 [74]
1477 (Couples)	SCL-90 Hostility Subscale, Self-reported behavior	Antisocial behavior moderately associated with relationship conflict	2012 [75]
112 (Couples)	DSM III-R	Men's ASPD predicted physical abuse, partner negative psychological adjustment and reduced marital satisfaction	1999, 2003 [76, 77]

Table 3. Relationship variables, marital adjustment and psychopathic personality traits in available studies to date.

of psychopathy, the behavior of many psychopathic individuals does not comport with this view. A survey of self-help message boards and clinical experience indicates that far more people are distressed by ongoing victimization and psychopathic individuals' refusal to sever ties than by psychopathic partner abandonment [45]. Stalking by psychopathic former partners is also reported [56]. Psychopathic individuals may become vindictive when threatened with abandonment even when they have been unfaithful [6, 57]. If vindictiveness, stalking, and/or refusal to sever ties is connected to a specific variant of psychopathy (perhaps secondary psychopathy), then the relative prevalence of this variant should be determined.

5.1. Do psychopathic individuals cultivate and remain in long-term romantic relationships?

One study of 1805 long-term married couples (average relationship length 19.6 years) found 49 (3%) women and 283 (16%) men reported three or more symptoms of APSD. Anecdotal reports also indicate that psychopathic individuals cultivate long-term romantic partnerships although infidelity is common [45, 47, 58]. Psychopathic individuals often con prospective partners by making misrepresentations regarding core aspects of their lives and identities. They then move the relationship along quickly, seeking early cohabitation and commitment [6, 45, 47, 58]. Partners meet in a variety of settings including through friends, work, place of worship, or school [58]. Passion is high early in the relationship when psychopathic individuals are noted to give material gifts and expressions of love and affection [58, 59]. Contrary to prevailing theory, partners report that even highly psychopathic individuals appear affectionate, especially in the beginning [47]. The beginning phase of the relationship can last several years depending on the circumstance and during this time, abuse is uncommon and the relationship may be harmonious [47]. In retrospect, partners can identify reasons why they were treated well in the beginning. Many say they were used as "cover" and that the psychopathic individual was trying to impress others or appear normal [45, 47, 58]. Others realize the motivation was parasitism. Pregnancy and childbirth are often the turning point where relationships become abusive. Boredom, infidelity, and escalation of substance use or gambling may also trigger partner abuse [60].

5.2. Is there a specific type of person who partners with a highly psychopathic individual?

There is evidence for assortative mating for psychopathic characteristics (see **Tables 3, 6–8**) [61–63]. Assortative mating may contribute significantly to intergenerational transmission [64]. Partner's personality type may be influenced by ACOA status as children of alcoholics may also tend to pair with psychopathic alcoholic individuals [65]. To test the hypothesis that women who partnered with psychopathic men might be temperamentally similar to their partners, the Temperament and Character Inventory was administered to a group of 35 women who were seeking support recovering from abusive relationships with psychopathic men. Narratives regarding the relationship were also collected from the women [58]. In common with psychopathic men, many women in the group had elevated Novelty Seeking scores. This elevation was due to Exploratory Excitability and not Impulsiveness, Extravagance or Disorderliness. In narrative accounts, many described being exhausted by the energy level of and chaos caused by their former partner. It may be that a certain need for excitement and tolerance for chaos is required by those who remain in a relationship with a highly psychopathic person. As one woman said, "It was the best and worst all rolled into one. I've never loved so much and in the same breath I've never hurt so much. Despite all his horrible qualities, he's still the most exciting person I've ever known (p. 86)." The women also had elevated scores in Reward Dependence, Cooperativeness, and Self-Determination, traits that would tend to facilitate a person remaining in (but also recovering from) an abusive relationship. In this and two other surveys of people seeking to recover from abusive relationships, participants identified their own vulnerabilities, including losses just prior to meeting the psychopathic partner and a history of child abuse or prior sexual assault [45].

5.3. Does psychopathy impact marital quality and relationship satisfaction?

There is little doubt that many psychopathic individuals are highly abusive of partners (see below). Partners who are not subjected to high levels of abuse are often distressed by sexual infidelity and financial concerns. In long-term partnerships, psychopathy is associated with marital dissatisfaction [18]. The Cambridge Study in Delinquent Development examined relationship satisfaction and durability longitudinally in men, some with high PCL-SV scores and criminal involvement. In this study, psychopathy was negatively associated with relationship satisfaction and this was attributable to high scores in the affective facet [66]. However, at age 48, most men were cohabitating with a female partner (82%) and endorsed (88%) "gets on well with female partner." These responses were not significantly associated with either criminality or psychopathy [67].

Twelve studies reveal a consistent negative influence of psychopathy on relationship quality (**Table 3**) [18, 59, 68–77]. Psychopathy is associated with reduced relationship satisfaction in both dating and cohabitating couples [59, 68]. Studies using the LSRP have found that secondary psychopathy impacts relationship quality more than primary psychopathy. The association between secondary psychopathy and decreased dyadic adjustment is not surprising, given high neuroticism and low conscientiousness in secondary psychopathy [71, 78] and the association between these and poor dyadic adjustment [71, 79]. Primary psychopathy is less robustly associated with low relationship satisfaction. In one study, primary psychopathy predicted a latent factor composed of passion, intimacy, and commitment [59]. Perhaps, individuals high in primary psychopathy are more adept at manipulating partners and using relationships for instrumental purposes [80]. The negative impact of psychopathy on well-being is mediated in part through poor quality of intimate relationships [68]. Turmoil in intimate relationships also predicts increases in self-reported psychopathy over time [71]. Poor parental dyadic adjustment also leads to increases in externalizing symptoms in children [18, 73–76, 81].

5.4. Is psychopathy associated with partner abuse?

Psychopathy underlies community violence including violence toward partners and friends [82]. DSM III-R links ASPD to "spouse or child beating" [54, p. 342]. Psychopathy is associated with intimate partner violence perpetration [83, 84] and intimate partner terrorism [85]. In intimate partner terrorism, all forms of abuse serve the purpose of coercive control of partners

http://dx.doi.org/10.5772/intechopen.70227

[86–88]. Psychopathic men and women's use of coercive control with partners is an extension of coercive familial behaviors learned during childhood and adolescence [34]. Learning of coercion occurs through both practice and modeling as witnessing domestic violence is a risk factor for the development of psychopathy [89]. Although some link coercive control to patriarchy [86], case histories of perpetrators suggest psychopathy [86, 90] and women perpetrate coercive control [87, 88]. It is likely that psychopathic personality traits associated with Factor 1 predispose to coercive control and also increase susceptibility to messages regarding patriarchy [91].

The extent to which psychopathy considered dimensionally is responsible for the public health problem of intimate partner violence has not been established. Certainly, the degree of psychopathy that increases risk for violence is far below that required for a categorical diagnosis [52]. In one study, abuse of partners was associated with psychopathy and this association was mediated by low Big Five Agreeableness [92]. Partners of psychopathic individuals endorse all forms of abuse including physical, sexual, psychological, emotional, social, financial, and legal [45]. The repercussions of financial abuse for victims have not been systematically investigated. Anecdotally, financial abuse causes poverty in middle age for people who otherwise would have been financially secure [42]. Interestingly, some highly psychopathic individuals contribute financially to their families [47]. Legal abuse occurs through the criminal court when psychopathic individuals recruit unwitting partners into their crimes and through civil court when partners attempt separation [6, 47]. Some psychopathic individuals are skilled at using the family courts to punish former partners [6, 93]. Social abuse occurs when psychopathic individuals spread rumors (a behavior victims have dubbed "the sociopath's smear campaign" [94]) or behave in ways that damage their partner's standing with others.

5.5. Couple therapy in the context of psychopathy

Couples present for couple therapy for reasons that "involve relational matters, such as emotional disengagement and waning commitment, power struggles, problem-solving and communication difficulties, jealousy and extramarital involvements, value and role conflicts, sexual dissatisfaction, and abuse and violence [95]"—all factors expected to be prevalent in the context of psychopathy. Given the association between psychopathy and relationship distress, this disorder is likely common in community couple therapy practice. Current guidelines stipulate that couple therapy not be offered to couples where: (1) the perpetrator of abuse lacks remorse, and does not take full responsibility for the abuse; (2) the perpetrator of abuse has a personality disorder; (3) the victim expresses fear; or (4) there is an ongoing threat of violence [96, 97]. Given that therapists are known not to adequately screen for these contraindications to couple therapy [98, 99], it is reasonable to hypothesize that many couples where these conditions are present do participate in couple therapy.

There are no published studies of couple therapy in the context of psychopathy or ASPD. In a preliminary study [60], 281 people (255 women, 26 men, all heterosexual) reporting relationships with a psychopathic partner (as assessed through DSM 5, Section III symptoms) answered an online survey regarding their experiences in couple therapy.

All participants reported psychological abuse and most reported multiple other forms of abuse including physical, financial, and sexual. Although open-ended survey responses describing relationship and partner characteristics clearly pointed to the presence of psychopathy, disorder was identified by a minority of therapists even when abuse was severe. Sixty-two percent of therapists appeared to participants to lack knowledge of psychopathy. Some therapists were reported to have learned about psychopathy only after interacting with the participant's partner. The combination of DSM 5, Section III Antagonism and Disinhibition symptoms, and therapist knowledge explained 60% of the variance in therapist identification of partner disorder. Therapist detection of partner symptoms was associated with the perceived helpfulness of treatment. One woman stated, "For the first time, someone wasn't manipulated by him to the point of thinking he was the victim instead of me. She called him on his 'red herrings' and got him back on track when he tried to talk about other things to pass the time." Participant responses indicated that couple therapists attempted the same communication exercises with them that are recommended for non-personality disordered couples (**Table 4**). Abused partners feel invalidated during these exercises that may also place them in danger [100]. Therapists who helped participants understand the nature of their partner's emotional deficits and manipulative behavior were judged most helpful. Only 11% of relationships continued; some therapists assisted participants in exiting the relationship. The responses of survey participants point to a gap in the literature that should be filled by more systematic investigation of community couple therapy practices.

5.6. Individual therapy for recovering partners of psychopathic individuals

At present, there are no evidence-supported interventions for partners or former partners of psychopathic individuals. A survey of 301 people, who had received individual psychotherapy for issues related to a long-term relationship with a psychopathic individual was conducted to determine interventions found most helpful and unhelpful by victims [101]. Also of interest was whether therapists were judged knowledgeable regarding the construct of psychopathy and the problem of psychopathy and the family. A minority of therapists were reported to have knowledge of psychopathy and its impact on the family. Participants reported invalidating responses, unhelpful, and harmful therapy when therapists lacked

Partner descriptions of communication exercises used in couple therapy
We were coached in active listener techniques, seeing the others point of view, using "I" statements and other non-aggressive communication strategies. The result was that my partner got better at communicating in a way that was manipulative, and he got better at making me feel guilty when I expressed the fact that I felt manipulated.
He wanted to soften me up and that was extremely unsafe to me. Using "I feel" was dangerous since husband would use those against me later. We had already been taught this communication years before but husband would never use the tools. Instead of listening to me, counselor would say "well done, you two!" like this was a major breakthrough. HUH? I often would confront him and ask why he was taking husband at face value (since he's a lying manipulator) He would come back with "well, how am I supposed to take him?" Well, maybe like an abuser????

Table 4. Example of open-ended response from two participants who described communication exercises used in couple therapy where partner had psychopathic personality traits.

knowledge of psychopathy. In open-ended and Likert responses, participants stated that understanding their former partner's personality disorder helped them make meaning of their experiences. Effective meaning making reduced self-blame and assisted in overcoming the distorted cognitions imparted to them by their abuser. Traditional approaches to family violence that attribute abuse to patriarchy as opposed to personality disorder may not be well suited for family members of psychopathic individuals. Such approaches do not assist with meaning making and risk of re-victimization related to pairing with another psychopathic individual. Furthermore, men victims of psychopathic partners require therapeutic assistance and do not fit the traditional model of domestic violence [88]. Former partners who share children with a psychopathic parent may not be able to cease having contact with their abuser. They need help learning effective strategies for dealing with the psychopathic co-parent (unfortunately, there are no data on effective strategies to provide them). These parents also need extensive support to provide the kind of nurturing parenting that will mitigate genetic risk for psychopathy [102].

6. Psychopathic parents

Parenting behavior and the family environment caused by psychopathic traits are important in the intergenerational transmission of psychopathy [103]. When I was trained in psychiatry, neglectful parenting behavior was part of the definition of ASPD in DSM III-R (**Table 4**) [54]. We were taught that people with ASPD neglect and abandon their children. In response to my presentations at scientific meetings, colleagues have opined that "psychopaths[2] [sic] are disinterested in parenting." Several years ago, I sat in family court observing a custody case regarding a father I knew to be highly psychopathic. The father paid a psychologist to testify on his behalf to rebut the neutral forensic evaluator who had diagnosed psychopathy. The paid expert testified that since this father wanted a relationship with his children, he could not be "a psychopath." The court transcript quotes the psychologist, "Robert Hare in his book says that psychopaths have no use for, or interest in children[3]…This man wants a relationship with his children and that is not typical for a psychopath." This belief may be firmly ingrained in mental health professionals and may be the reason why parenting in relation to psychopathy is understudied. As with romantic partners, the problem of psychopathy and parenting is not abandonment [105]. It is psychopathic parents' motivation to maintain ties with children who they neglect, abuse, and expose to antisocial activities.

6.1. Studies of parenting behavior in people with psychopathic traits

A comprehensive list of studies of paternal [103, 105–115], maternal [116–122], and parental [73, 75, 93, 123–126] behavior in relation to psychopathic traits is provided in **Tables 6–8**. There

[2]It is not within ethical guidelines to refer to a person by their diagnosis. The use of particular cut points for diagnosis of categorical psychopathy has not been adequately justified.
[3]Dr. Hare (with whom I shared this story) did not say this in *Without Conscience* [104], nor does he endorse the statement of this psychologist. *Without Conscience* (p. 63) clearly states that psychopathic parents often claim to love their children, even when they neglect and abuse them.

is one large-scale study of parenting and psychopathic traits [123]. Dimensional Psychopathy correlates with reduced closeness, parenting stress, and unhappiness with the parenting role (**Table 6**). The three parenting studies that examined the correlation between paternal and maternal psychopathic traits found small to moderate correlations [107, 110, 126]. Psychopathy in fathers is associated with abandonment and IPV perpetration, especially in the context of maternal psychopathic features [110, 125, 126]. Outcome for children is worse when antisocial fathers maintain contact [105, 107, 110, 111, 127]. Psychopathic traits are associated with coercive, hostile and neglectful fathering, and low warmth. Paternal psychopathy impacts the structure of children's lives due to poor marital quality, unstable housing, a chaotic home environment, and poverty [103]. Maternal psychopathy is associated with lower age at first birth [109, 125]. Regardless of age, psychopathic mothers may be abusive and neglectful, and show inappropriately low levels of monitoring and inconsistent discipline; their mothering tends to be hostile, coercive, and shaming with low levels of warmth (**Tables 5** and **6**). Outcome for children is related to the home environment and parenting practices of psychopathic mothers [117, 119, 120]. There are no studies examining whether there is a dose-effect of exposure to psychopathic mothers as there is with psychopathic fathers with respect to negative outcome.

Anecdotal reports and qualitative studies provide first-hand accounts of the human suffering caused by parental psychopathy [6, 93]. Children and adults describe a confusing combination of loving and abusive experiences; this mix of experiences and the trauma associated with parental psychopathy produces disorganized attachment and dissociation of parental object representations [64, 83]. Children (who often carry genetic risk [105]) may develop internalizing and/or externalizing disorders. Psychopathic parents may select both favorites and targets for abuse from among the children of the family [93]. Favorites are overindulged and provided lax supervision, while targets are subjected to shaming and other abuse [93]. Psychopathic parents may enjoy inducing fear in their children and they may maintain poor sexual boundaries [93]. Psychoticism, defined as unusual beliefs and experiences, eccentricity, and perceptual dysregulation (DSM 5, Section III) is apparent in descriptions of parents provided by adult offspring and former partners [45, 47, 58, 93]; psychoticism manifests in the psychopathic individuals' distorted worldview. The family takes on "cult-like" characteristics when psychopathic individuals demand that family members endorse their distorted views and unusual beliefs [93].

Parenting behavior diagnostic of antisocial personality disorder (ASPD)
(4) repeatedly fails to honor financial obligations, as indicated by defaulting on debts or failing to provide child support or support other dependents on a regular basis.
(8) if a parent or guardian, lacks ability to function as a responsible parent, as indicated by one or more of the following:
(a) malnutrition of child
(b) child's illness resulting from lack of minimal hygiene
(c) failure to obtain medical care for a seriously ill child
(d) child's dependence on neighbors or nonresident relatives for food or shelter
(e) failure to arrange for a caretaker of a young child when parent is away from home
(f) repeated squandering, on personal items, of money required for household necessities

Table 5. Parenting behavior in DSM III-R criteria for antisocial personality disorder.

Studies of Psychopathy and Fathering			
N	**Definition of psychopathic traits**	**Study Findings**	**Study Publication year [Reference]**
478	PCL-SV	Paternal psychopathy linked to unstable employment, unstable housing and substance abuse, and psychopathy in offspring	2015 [103]
34 ASPD+/SD+	SCID II; DSM III-R ASPD	Children of ASPD+/SD+ fathers had higher externalizing and internalizing psychopathology and association with deviant peers than both ASPD−/SD+ and ASPD−/SD−.	2002 [106]
161	SCID II; DSM IV ASPD	ASPD associated with paternal abandonment. ASPD in mother and father correlated.	2001 [107]
20	PSCAN; Partner report	Children exposed to IPV; father abused children by lying to them, ignoring them, failing to provide for them, bullying and terrifying them, breaking promises to them, and destroying their toys	2005 [108]
1116	DSM IV ASPD	"When fathers engaged in high levels of antisocial behavior, the more time they lived with their children, the more conduct problems their children had"	2003 [105]
980	DSM IV CD	CD was associated with earlier age at first birth, IPV, negative parenting practices and DBDs in children	2006 [109]
1626	DSM III-R	Mother and father ASB correlated. Mother ASB negatively correlated with father residence. Father ASB correlated with non-residence. Child behavior problems increased with amount of time with father. "As the length of time that the father was present in the home increased, so too did the strength of the relationship between father and child antisocial behavior"	2008 [110]
230	MMPI-TRI *Agreeableness* subscale from the NEO-Five factor inventory	Child behavior problems were associated with more time spent with antisocial fathers. Coercive fathering was predicted by antisocial personality features in fathers	2010 [111]
261	ASB	ASB was associated with harsh discipline and low warmth. ASB associated with internalizing and externalizing symptoms that increased with the amount of contact between father and child	2011 [112]
543	ASB	Father-child contact mediates intergenerational continuity of ASB, effect mediated by dysfunctional parenting	2009 [113]
96	Antisocial behavior	Antisocial fathers with alcohol use disorders, family shows less engagement during interactions	2000 [128]
145	PDQ-4 ASPD	Paternal ASPD and Borderline PD traits were correlated; ASPD traits correlated with psychological and physical aggression and predicted children's overall psychosocial impairment and externalizing problems	2014 [13]
8	IPV perpetration	Qualitative study of children's lived experience. Children observed to dissociate. Had difficulty integrating conflicting observations of and feelings toward father. Children felt "trapped in conflict" and responsible for father's "influence"	2015 [14]
66	IPV perpetration	Greater contact with father, more externalizing problems and more exposure to IPV	2016 [15]

Table 6. Parenting behavior and child outcomes for psychopathic fathers.

An examination of the complete quantitative and qualitative literature reveals consistent patterns in the relations between children's experiences and the construct of parental psychopathy (**Figure 1**). Although most quantitative studies assessed primarily traits related to PCL-R Factor 2, there is sufficient evidence to conclude that Factor 1 traits also impact parenting and determine children's experience. Pathological lying and the other interpersonal manifestations of psychopathy link to severe emotional and psychological abuse [93]. Invalidation and "gas-lighting" cause children to doubt their own perceptions of reality. Parental alienation (parental attempts to distance the child from a loving co-parent) may be one manifestation of "gas-lighting" [6]. Affective deficits and dominance needs cause parents to enjoy frightening and shaming children. Parents' affective deficits produce guilt and confusion and impair trust [6, 93]. Lifestyle deficits cause unstable residence, neglect, and poverty [103] (see **Tables 6–8**). Early behavioral problems and juvenile delinquency may be markers for increased genetic risk in children. Criminal behavior and poor behavioral controls cause modeling of antisocial behavior, coercive control and physical abuse. The sexual symptoms of psychopathy cause exposure to multiple (perhaps psychopathic) stepparents, exposure to sexually inappropriate material, and sexual abuse [93].

6.2. Assessment of children and custody recommendations

The clinical literature and the family courts may refer to couples where there is an abusive psychopathic parent and a victimized partner as "high conflict" [75, 128, 129]. Child victims

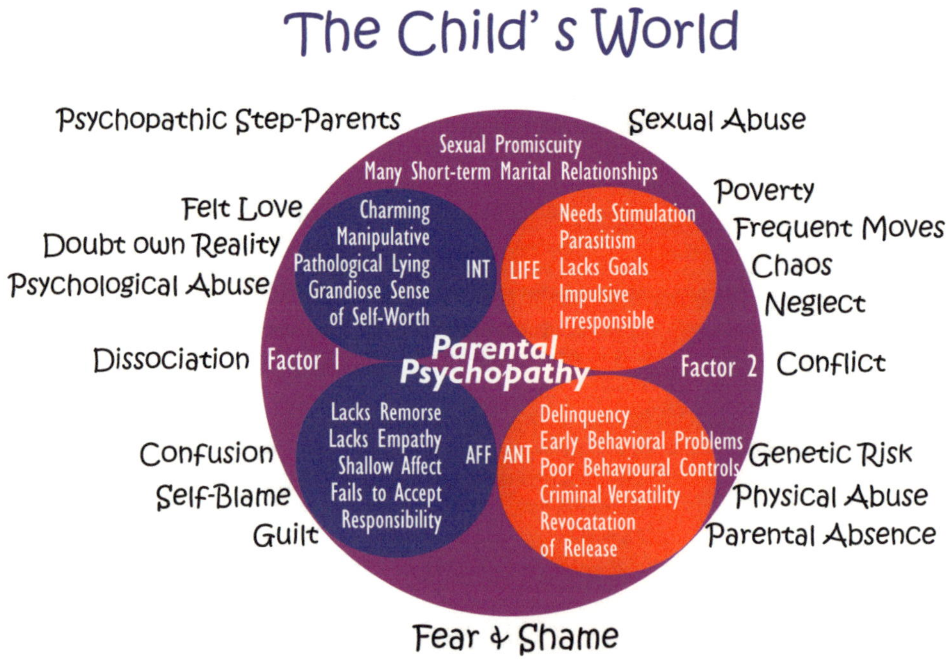

Figure 1. The relationship between parental psychopathy and children's lived experience. Symptoms of psychopathy are in the center of the circle, Factor 1 [Interpersonal (INT), Affective (AFF)] symptoms are on the left; Factor 2 [Lifestyle (LIFE), Antisocial (ANT)] are on the right, sexual symptoms are on top. Children's lived experience is portrayed in Kristen ITC font in the outer circle adjacent to associated facets. Fear and shame are central to the experience of having a psychopathic parent.

Studies of Psychopathy and Mothering			
N	**Definition of psychopathic traits**	**Study Findings**	**Study Publication Year [Reference]**
141	MMPI-2 ASP Scale	Pd scale of MMPI had poor predictive validity with respect to parenting measures. ASP scale antisocial mothers less understanding, more abusive, used shame, and coercion	2014 [123]
1116	DSM IV ASPD	ASPD mothers' home environment poor; chaotic; reduced happiness, reduced stimulation, parenting stress; ASPD mothers had less positive parenting less warmth and more negativity. Child neglect present in 16.2% ASPD only and 33.9% ASPD/Depression	2012 [124]
88	PPI-R; PDQ-4	ASPD symptoms linked to poor monitoring, inconsistent discipline, decreased involvement, boys' CU, impulsive and narcissistic traits	2012 [125]
83	LSRP	Primary and secondary psychopathy associated with parenting dysfunction and child conduct problems	2013 [129]
201	C-DIS-IV (DSM IV)	Maternal ASPD associated with IPV exposure and child DBDs. Maternal ASPD not associated with parenting indices, impact of dysfunctional parenting mediated by IPV exposure and child temperament	2010 [126]
299	Adult Self Report (ASR)	Maternal ASB associated with depression, hostile parenting, and child DBDs	2012 [75]
126	Family Informant Schedule and Criteria (FISC)	Maternal ASB associated with poor monitoring; maternal CD associated with decreased punishment; other parenting variables not associated with either ASB or CD	2013 [93]

Table 7. Parenting behavior and child outcomes for psychopathic mothers.

are conceptualized as being caught up in "parental conflict" rather than in a situation where one parent has the burden of protecting them from abuse [130]. Such terminology conveys the impression that the non-psychopathic victimized co-parent is partly responsible for the family pathology. Although psychopathy in mothers and fathers is correlated, correlations are modest. Professionals involved with the family should therefore assess psychopathy dimensions in both partners using all available data. Evaluators should carefully consider the credibility of information they are given. If psychopathic traits are suspected, evaluators should document the presence of symptoms from all four facets of psychopathy and consider the differential impact of these on the child (**Figure 1**). The presence of mood, anxiety, and substance use disorders in parents should be assessed. Domestic violence including all forms of partner and child abuse should be documented. Clinicians should attempt to classify the family according to whether psychopathy is significant in one or both parents and as to whether abuse is primarily unidirectional. There are sufficient data (**Tables 6–8**) to recommend that if there is a relatively healthy parent, contact with the psychopathic parent should be limited. For further discussion of custody evaluations, see Refs. [5] and [6].

Relatively healthy parents should be referred for treatment of problems associated with any trauma they may have suffered. They should also be counseled regarding the detrimental impact disordered stepparents might have on children. The risk for revictimization by another psychopathic partner should be discussed. There are no data as to the frequency with which

Studies of Psychopathy and Parenting			
N	**Definition of psychopathic traits**	**Study Findings**	**Study Publication year [Reference]**
15,701	Big 5 facets associated with psychopathy	Reduced happiness with the parenting role; reduced closeness; increased stress from children; overwhelmed with role	2014 [123]
145	IPDE-S	ASPD symptoms associated with lower quality responsiveness by mothers and child attempts to engage parent in social interaction. NPD symptoms associated with controlling parenting in both mothers and fathers	2012 [124]
99 mothers 72 fathers	ASB, arrest records and self-report	3-generation study, mother and father ASB correlated; father ASB negatively correlated with contact with child; ASB in mother correlated with younger age of first birth	2012 [125]
1255	DSM–III–R ASPD	Antisocial parents had significantly lower levels of cohesion and satisfaction, lower consensus on important issues, and a lower overall marital quality. Antisocial mothers and fathers dysfunctional parenting; fathers less involved	2013 [128]
489	DSM IV ASPD	ASB in mother and father correlated. ASB correlated with adversity for children, parental neglect, and exposure to violence	2010 [126]
1477	Antisocial behavior	Antisocial mothers and fathers more hostile parenting, these related to child ASB	2012 [75]
9	PCL-R, DSM 5	Qualitative study; psychopathic parents can be granted custody; psychopathy associated with abuse, neglect, exposure to multiple antisocial adults, chaotic home environment, unstable residence, poverty; children report: fear, confusion, shame, and anger; some given false information regarding their identity; children also report positive family experiences and feelings of love and loyalty toward psychopathic parent; family resembles a "cult"	2013 [93]

Table 8. Parenting behavior and child outcomes for psychopathic fathers and mothers.

children are forced to spend time with or are placed by the courts in the custody of abusive psychopathic parents. My clinical experience and anecdotal evidence suggest this may be a serious problem in all Western democracies [93]. Professionals can assist children who have been victimized by recommending to the court that they be given truthful information as they can tolerate it (to counteract pathological lying and gas-lighting). Children may do better if the relatively healthy parent is coached as to how to provide them with direct truthful answers to questions [128] (although some localities have laws that prohibit parents from answering children's questions truthfully [93]). Professionals should be aware of the possibility that if there is a marital separation, children may be jeopardized by a court decision to grant unsupervised parenting time to a psychopathic parent. Circumstances may dictate that a co-parent remain in an abusive relationship to protect (a) young child(ren).

7. Family involvement in the treatment of psychopathy

Studies of families, relationship quality, conflict, and psychopathy show that marital problems and parent child problems worsen symptoms of psychopathy in mothers, fathers, sons, and daughters (**Tables 3** and **6–8**). Families may thus get caught in a positive feedback loop of worsening relations and psychopathic features. If therapy could reduce conflict and enhance relationship quality, symptoms of psychopathy in family members would likely decline. Evidence supported family therapy for adult psychopathy has not been developed though family therapies for adolescents with externalizing disorders do exist [131]. Studies of family therapy for youth with externalizing disorders should assess parental psychopathy to assess its impact on treatment effectiveness. Psychopathy is known to be a poor prognostic indicator for batterer intervention [132].

Anecdotal reports note that some family members assist psychopathic individuals in evading arrest and capture and others hold them accountable [47, 93]. Forensic experts report that marriage reduces criminal recidivism in psychopathic individuals [133]. In the case of "Frank" mentioned in the Introduction, the treating clinician stated, "Frank's wife has indicated that she is invested in Frank's recovery and remains connected to him. Her willingness to support his recovery should be explored. The possibility of a pharmacologic intervention may encourage her to remain supportive, *given her forgiving nature* (p. 190, emphasis added)." There are no studies that assess the relative societal benefit of spousal support in preventing recidivism in the context of detriments to the health and well-being of the marriage partner or children. I did study one case of a wife and mother who endured years of abuse at the hands of her psychopathic husband to protect her daughter and other women from rape. Her relief came only when her husband was convicted and jailed with her assistance [47, 134]. I could not locate a discussion of the ethical issues raised when clinicians encourage spouses and other family members to remain connected to psychopathic individuals.

8. Summary

Psychopathy is clearly a familial disorder and a disorder of the family. Dysfunctional family relationships both worsen and are worsened by psychopathy. The long-standing belief that psychopathic individuals do not form lasting bonds with others has hindered therapeutic progress. While the nature of social reward for highly psychopathic individuals is yet to be determined, they do not prefer to be solitary. Forensic and community studies reveal that most psychopathic individuals maintain social ties over years and that these ties serve their psychological and material needs. Taken in its entirety, the psychopathy literature suggests that dominance reward [19] from both social power and material resource control [20] motivates sociability for highly psychopathic individuals. Couple and family therapy for psychopathy should be studied in the context of disorder severity. Also needed are evidence supported therapies for recovering adult sons and daughters and former partners of psychopathic persons.

Author details

Liane J. Leedom

Address all correspondence to: lleedom@bridgeport.edu

University of Bridgeport, Bridgeport, Connecticut, USA

References

[1] Brody Y, Rosenfeld B. Object relations in criminal psychopaths. International Journal of Offender Therapy and Comparative Criminology. 2002 Aug;**46**(4):400-411

[2] Eisenman R. Living with a psychopathic personality: Case history of a successful antisocial personality. Acta Paedopsychiatrica: International Journal of Child and Adolescent Psychiatry. 1993 Apr;**56**(1):53-55

[3] Krupp DB, Sewall LA, Lalumière ML, Sheriff C, Harris GT. Nepotistic patterns of violent psychopathy: Evidence for adaptation? Frontiers in Psychology. 2012;**3**:305

[4] DeLisi M. Psychopathy is the unified theory of crime. Youth Violence and Juvenile Justice. 2009 Jul 1;**7**(3):256-273

[5] Felthous A, Sass H. International Handbook on Psychopathic Disorders and the Law. West Sussex, England, UK: John Wiley & Sons; 2012

[6] Häkkänen-Nyholm H, Nyholm J-O. Psychopathy and Law: A Practitioner's Guide. West Sussex, England, UK: John Wiley & Sons; 2012

[7] Patrick CJ. Handbook of Psychopathy. New York, NY: Guilford Press; 2005. p. 673

[8] Glenn AL, Raine A. Psychopathy: An Introduction to Biological Findings and their Implications. New York, NY: NYU Press; 2014

[9] Salekin RT, Lynam DR. Handbook of Child and Adolescent Psychopathy. New York, NY: Guilford Press; 2011

[10] Gacono CB. The Clinical and Forensic Assessment of Psychopathy: A Practitioner's Guide. New York, NY: Routledge; 2015

[11] Millon T, Simonsen E, Birket-Smith M, Davis RD. Psychopathy: Antisocial, Criminal, and Violent Behavior. New York, NY: Guilford Press; 2003

[12] Cleckley HM. The Mask of Sanity: An Attempt to Clarify Some Issues About the So-called Psychopathic Personality. St. Louis, MO: C. V. Mosby Co.; 1964. p. 520

[13] Rotgers F, Maniacci M. Antisocial Personality Disorder: A Practitioner's Guide to Comparative Treatments. New York, NY: Springer Publishing Company; 2005. p. 226

[14] National Collaborating Centre for Mental Health (UK). Antisocial Personality Disorder: Treatment, Management and Prevention [Internet]. Leicester (UK): British Psychological

Society; 2010. (National Institute for Health and Clinical Excellence: Guidance). Available from: http://www.ncbi.nlm.nih.gov/books/NBK55345/ [Accessed: April 26, 2017]

[15] Compton WM, Conway KP, Stinson FS, Colliver JD, Grant BF. Prevalence, correlates, and comorbidity of DSM-IV antisocial personality syndromes and alcohol and specific drug use disorders in the United States: Results from the national epidemiologic survey on alcohol and related conditions. The Journal of Clinical Psychiatry. 2005 Jun;**66**(6):677-685

[16] Coid J, Yang M, Ullrich S, Roberts A, Hare RD. Prevalence and correlates of psychopathic traits in the household population of Great Britain. International Journal of Law and Psychiatry. 2009 Mar;**32**(2):65-73

[17] U.S. Census Bureau. Annual Estimates of the Resident Population: April 1, 2010 to July 1, 2014 [Internet]. 2015. Available from: http://factfinder.census.gov/faces/tableservices/jsf/pages/productview.xhtml?src=bkmk

[18] Humbad MN, Donnellan MB, Iacono WG, Burt SA. Externalizing psychopathology and marital adjustment in long-term marriages: Results from a large combined sample of married couples. Journal of Abnormal Psychology. 2010 Feb;**119**(1):151

[19] Johnson SL, Leedom LJ, Muhtadie L. The dominance behavioral system and psychopathology: Evidence from self-report, observational, and biological studies. Psychological Bulletin. 2012 Apr 16;**138**(4):692-743

[20] Hawley PH. Social dominance in childhood and adolescence: Why social competence and aggression may go hand in hand. In: Aggression and Adaptation: The Bright Side to Bad Behavior [Internet]. Mahwah, NJ, US: Lawrence Erlbaum Associates Publishers; 2007. pp. 1-29. Available from: http://search.ebscohost.com/login.aspx?direct=true&db=psyh&AN=2007-07567-001&site=ehost-live

[21] Patterson GR, Stouthamer-Loeber M. The correlation of family management practices and delinquency. Child Development. 1984;**55**(4):1299-1307

[22] Hawes DJ, Dadds MR, Frost ADJ, Hasking PA. Do childhood callous-unemotional traits drive change in parenting practices? Journal of Clinical Child & Adolescent Psychology. 2011 Jul;**40**(4):507-518

[23] Ge X, Conger RD, Cadoret RJ, Neiderhiser JM, Yates W, Troughton E, et al. The developmental interface between nature and nurture: A mutual influence model of child antisocial behavior and parent behaviors. Developmental Psychology. 1996 Jul;**32**(4):574-589

[24] Rhee SH, Waldman ID. Genetic and environmental influences on antisocial behavior: A meta-analysis of twin and adoption studies. Psychological Bulletin. 2002 May;**128**(3):490-529

[25] Dishion TJ, Stormshak EA, Kavanagh KA. Everyday Parenting: A Professional's Guide to Building Family Management Skills. Champaign, IL, US: Research Press; 2012

[26] McDonald R, Dodson MC, Rosenfield D, Jouriles EN. Effects of a parenting intervention on features of psychopathy in children. Journal of Abnormal Child Psychology. 2011 Oct;**39**(7):1013-1023

[27] Livingston G. Family size among mothers [Internet]. Pew Research Center's Social & Demographic Trends Project. 2015. Available from: http://www.pewsocialtrends.org/2015/05/07/family-size-among-mothers/ [Accessed: April 26, 2017]

[28] Eurostat. Families by Type, Size and NUTS 3 Region – Eurostat [Internet]. 2016. Available from: http://ec.europa.eu/eurostat/web/products-datasets/-/cens_11fts_r3 [Accessed: May 9, 2017]

[29] Pike, A. Commentary: Are siblings birds of a feather? – reflections on Jenkins et al. Journal of Child Psychology and Psychiatry. 2012; **53**:630-631. DOI:10.1111/j.1469-7610.2012.02536.x

[30] Krienert JL, Walsh JA. Sibling sexual abuse: An empirical analysis of offender, victim, and event characteristics in National Incident-Based Reporting System (NIBRS) data, 2000-2007. Journal of Child Sexual Abuse: Research, Treatment, & Program Innovations for Victims, Survivors, & Offenders. 2011 Jul;**20**(4):353-372

[31] Khan R, Cooke DJ. Risk factors for severe inter-sibling violence: A preliminary study of a youth forensic sample. Journal of Interpersonal Violence. 2008 Feb 28;**23**(11):1513-1530

[32] Patterson GR. Siblings: Fellow travelers in coercive family processes. Advances in the Study of Aggression. 1984;**1**:173-215

[33] Snyder J, Bank L, Burraston B. The consequences of antisocial behavior in older male siblings for younger brothers and sisters. Journal of Family Psychology. 2005 Dec;**19**(4):643-653

[34] Shortt JW, Capaldi DM, Dishion TJ, Bank L, Owen LD. The role of adolescent friends, romantic partners, and siblings in the emergence of the adult antisocial lifestyle. Journal of Family Psychology. 2003 Dec;**17**(4):521-533

[35] Kosson DS, Blackburn R, Byrnes KA, Park S, Logan C, Donnelly JP. Assessing interpersonal aspects of schizoid personality disorder: Preliminary validation studies. Journal of Personality Assessment. 2008 Mar;**90**(2):185-196

[36] Dupéré V, Lacourse É, Willms JD, Vitaro F, Tremblay RE. Affiliation to youth gangs during adolescence: The interaction between childhood psychopathic tendencies and neighborhood disadvantage. Journal of Abnormal Child Psychology. 2007 Dec;**35**(6):1035-1045

[37] Valdez A, Kaplan CD, Codina E. Psychopathy among Mexican American gang members: A comparative study. International Journal of Offender Therapy and Comparative Criminology. 2000 Feb;**44**(1):46-58

[38] Sherretts N, Boduszek D, Debowska A. Exposure to criminal environment and criminal social identity in a sample of adult prisoners: The moderating role of psychopathic traits. Law and Human Behavior. 2016 Aug;**40**(4):430-439

[39] Goldweber A, Dmitrieva J, Cauffman E, Piquero AR, Steinberg L. The development of criminal style in adolescence and young adulthood: Separating the lemmings from the loners. Journal of Youth and Adolescence. 2011 Mar;**40**(3):332-346

[40] Williams TF, Thomas KM, Donnellan MB, Hopwood CJ. The aversive interpersonal behaviors associated with pathological personality traits. Journal of Personality Disorders. 2014 Dec;**28**(6):824-840

[41] Foulkes L, Seara-Cardoso A, Neumann CS, Rogers JSC, Viding E. Looking after number one: Associations between psychopathic traits and measures of social motivation and functioning in a community sample of males. Journal of Psychopathology and Behavioral Assessment. 2014 Mar;**36**(1):22-29

[42] Muñoz LC, Kerr M, Besic N. The peer relationships of youths with psychopathic personality traits: A matter of perspective. Criminal Justice and Behavior. 2008 Feb;**35**(2):212-227

[43] Maaß U, Lämmle L, Bensch D, Ziegler M. Narcissists of a feather flock together: Narcissism and the similarity of friends. Personality and Social Psychology Bulletin. 2016 Mar;**42**(3):366-384

[44] Baird SA. The links between primary and secondary psychopathy and social adaptation. Colgate University Journal of the Sciences. 2002;**34**:61-82

[45] Leedom LJ, Andersen D. Antisocial/Psychopathic Personality: What do Family Members, Romantic Partners and Friends Report? In: Society for the Scientific Study of Psychopathy Program (SSSP '11); 19-21 May, 2011, Montreal, Canada, 2011; p. 21

[46] University of Southern California. ScienceDaily. USC Study Finds Faulty Wiring in Psychopaths [Internet]. Available from: https://www.sciencedaily.com/releases/2004/03/040311072248.htm [Accessed: April 27, 2017]

[47] Leedom LJ, Geislin E, Hartoonian Almas L. "Did he ever love me?" A qualitative study of life with a psychopathic husband. Family & Intimate Partner Violence Quarterly. 2013;**5**(2):103-135

[48] Decker SH, Curry GD. Gangs, gang homicides, and gang loyalty: Organized crimes or disorganized criminals. Journal of Criminal Justice. 2002 Jul;**30**(4):343-352

[49] De Brito SA, Viding E, Kumari V, Blackwood N, Hodgins S. Cool and hot executive function impairments in violent offenders with antisocial personality disorder with and without psychopathy [Internet]. PLoS One. 2013 Jun 20;**8**(6) e65566

[50] Mathieu C, Neumann C, Babiak P, Hare RD. Corporate psychopathy and the full-range leadership model. Assessment. 2015;**22**(3):267-278

[51] Mathieu C, Babiak P. Corporate psychopathy and abusive supervision: Their influence on employees' job satisfaction and turnover intentions. Personality and Individual Differences. 2016 Mar;**91**:102-106

[52] Babiak P, Hare RD. Snakes in Suits: When Psychopaths Go to Work [Internet]. New York, NY, US: Regan Books/Harper Collins Publishers; 2006. Available from: http://search.ebscohost.com/login.aspx?direct=true&db=psyh&AN=2006-08313-000&site=ehost-live

[53] Hare RD, Neumann CS. Manual for the Revised Psychopathy Checklist. 2nd ed. Toronto, Canada: Multi Health Systems; 2003

[54] American Psychiatric Association. Diagnostic and Statistical Manual of Mental Health Disorders (DSM-III-R). American Psychiatric Association; 1987

[55] Jonason PK, Kavanagh P. The dark side of love: Love styles and the Dark Triad. Personality and Individual Differences. 2010 Oct;**49**(6):606-610

[56] Reavis JA, Allen EK, Meloy JR. Psychopathy in a mixed gender sample of adult stalkers. Journal of the Forensic Science. 2008 Sep;**53**(5):1214-1217

[57] Brewer G, Hunt D, James G, Abell L. Dark triad traits, infidelity and romantic revenge. Personality and Individual Differences. 2015;**83**:122-127

[58] Brown S, Leedom LJ. Women Who Love Psychopaths. Fairfield, CT: Health and Well-Being Publications; 2008. p. 120

[59] Ali F, Chamorro-Premuzic T. The dark side of love and life satisfaction: Associations with intimate relationships, psychopathy and Machiavellianism. Personality and Individual Differences. 2010 Jan;**48**(2):228-233

[60] Leedom LJ, Andersen D, Glynn MA. Couple therapy and intimate partner violence: A mixed methods study of victim experiences. Submitt Publ. 2017

[61] Krueger RF, Moffitt TE, Caspi A, Bleske A, Silva PA. Assortative mating for antisocial behavior: Developmental and methodological implications. Behavior Genetics. 1998 May;**28**(3):173-186

[62] Boutwell BB, Beaver KM, Barnes JC. More alike than different assortative mating and antisocial propensity in adulthood. Criminal Justice Review. 2012 Sep 1;**39**(9):1240-1254

[63] Moffitt TE, Caspi A, Rutter M, Silva PA. Sex Differences in Antisocial Behaviour: Conduct Disorder, Delinquency, and Violence in the Dunedin Longitudinal Study. New York, NY, US: Cambridge University Press; 2001

[64] Maes HH, Silberg JL, Neale MC, Eaves LJ. Genetic and cultural transmission of antisocial behavior: An extended twin parent model. Twin Research and Human Genetics: The Official Journal of the International Society for Twin Studies. 2007 Feb;**10**(1):136-150

[65] Schuckit MA, Tipp JE, Kelner E. Are daughters of alcoholics more likely to marry alcoholics? American Journal of Drug and Alcohol Abuse. 1994 May;**20**(2):237-245

[66] Ullrich S, Farrington DP, Coid JW. Psychopathic personality traits and life-success. Personality and Individual Differences. 2008 Apr;**44**(5):1162-1171

[67] Farrington DP, Coid JW, Harnett L, Jolliffe D, Soteriou N, Turner R, et al. Findings 281 [Internet]. 2006. Available from: http://www.crim.cam.ac.uk/people/academic_research/david_farrington/hofind281.pdf [Accessed: April 30, 2017]

[68] Love AB, Holder MD. Can romantic relationship quality mediate the relation between psychopathy and subjective well-being? Journal of Happiness Studies. 2016 Dec 1;**17**(6):2407-2429

[69] Smith CV, Hadden BW, Webster GD, Jonason PK, Gesselman AN, Crysel LC. Mutually attracted or repulsed? Actor–partner interdependence models of Dark Triad traits and relationship outcomes. Personality and Individual Differences. 2014;**67**:35-41

[70] Savard C, Sabourin S, Lussier Y. Male sub-threshold psychopathic traits and couple distress. Personality and Individual Differences. 2006 Apr;**40**(5):931-942

[71] Savard C, Sabourin S, Lussier Y. Correlates of psychopathic personality traits in community couples. Personality and Mental Health. 2011;**5**(3):186-199

[72] Savard C, Brassard A, Lussier Y, Sabourin S. Subclinical psychopathic traits and romantic attachment in community couples: A dyadic approach. Personality and Individual Differences. 2015;**72**:128-134

[73] Bornovalova MA, Cummings JR, Hunt E, Blazei R, Malone S, Iacono WG. Understanding the relative contributions of direct environmental effects and passive genotype–environment correlations in the association between familial risk factors and child disruptive behavior disorders. Psychological Medicine. 2014 Mar;**44**(4):831-844

[74] Meyer JM, Rutter M, Silberg JL, Maes HH, Simonoff E, Shillady LL, et al. Familial aggregation for conduct disorder symptomatology: The role of genes, marital discord and family adaptability. Psychological Medicine. 2000 Jul;**30**(4):759-774

[75] Harold GT, Elam KK, Lewis G, Rice F, Thapar A. Interparental conflict, parent psychopathology, hostile parenting, and child antisocial behavior: Examining the role of maternal versus paternal influences using a novel genetically sensitive research design. Development and Psychopathology. 2012 Nov;**24**(4):1283-1295

[76] Fals-Stewart W, Birchler GR, O'Farrell TJ. Drug-abusing patients and their intimate partners: Dyadic adjustment, relationship stability, and substance use. Journal of Abnormal Psychology. 1999 Feb;**108**(1):11-23

[77] Fals-Stewart W, Kelley ML, Cooke CG, Golden JC. Predictors of the psychosocial adjustment of children living in households of parents in which fathers abuse drugs: The effects of postnatal parental exposure. Addictive Behaviors. 2003 Aug;**28**(6):1013-1031

[78] Salekin RT, Chen DR, Sellbom M, Lester WS, MacDougall E. Examining the factor structure and convergent and discriminant validity of the levenson self-report psychopathy scale: Is the two-factor model the best fitting model? Personality Disorders: Theory, Research, and Treatment. 2014 Jul;**5**(3):289-304

[79] Gattis KS, Berns S, Simpson LE, Christensen A. Birds of a feather or strange birds? Ties among personality dimensions, similarity, and marital quality. Journal of Family Psychology. 2004 Dec;**18**(4):564-574

[80] Colwell JT. An interpersonal method for scoring the tat: Implications for distinguishing individuals with psychopathic symptomatology using leary's circumplex model [Doctoral Dissertation]. US: Rosalind Franklin University; 1998

[81] Fals-Stewart W, Leonard KE, Birchler GR. The occurrence of male-to-female intimate partner violence on days of men's drinking: The moderating effects of antisocial personality disorder. Journal of Consulting and Clinical Psychology. 2005 Apr;**73**(2):239-248

[82] Coid J, Yang M. The impact of psychopathy on violence among the household population of Great Britain. Social Psychiatry and Psychiatric Epidemiology. 2011 Jun;**46**(6):473-480

[83] Harris GT, Hilton NZ, Rice ME. Explaining the frequency of intimate partner violence by male perpetrators: Do attitude, relationship, and neighborhood variables add to antisociality? Social Psychiatry and Psychiatric Epidemiology. 2011 Apr;**38**(4):309-331

[84] Huss MT, Covell CN, Langhinrichsen-Rohling J. Clinical implications for the assessment and treatment of antisocial and psychopathic domestic violence perpetrators. Journal of Aggression, Maltreatment & Trauma. 2006;**13**(1):59-85

[85] Johnson MP. A Typology of Domestic Violence: Intimate Terrorism, Violent Resistance, and Situational Couple Violence. UPNE; 2010. p. 175

[86] Stark E. Coercive Control: How Men Entrap Women in Personal Life. New York, NY, US: Oxford University Press; 2007. (Interpersonal violence)

[87] Tanha M, Beck CJA, Figueredo AJ, Raghavan C. Sex differences in intimate partner violence and the use of coercive control as a motivational factor for intimate partner violence. Journal of Interpersonal Violence. 2010 Oct;**25**(10):1836-1854

[88] Straus MA, Gozjolko KL. "Intimate Terrorism" and gender differences in injury of dating partners by male and female university students. Journal of Family Violence. 2014;**29**(1):51-65

[89] Dargis M, Koenigs M. Witnessing domestic violence during childhood is associated with psychopathic traits in adult male criminal offenders. Law and Human Behavior. 2017 Apr;**41**(2):173-179

[90] Bancroft L, Silverman JG, Ritchie D. The Batterer as Parent: Addressing the Impact of Domestic Violence on Family Dynamics. Thousand Oaks, CA, US: SAGE Publications; 2011. p. 353

[91] LeBreton JM, Baysinger MA, Abbey A, Jacques-Tiura AJ. The relative importance of psychopathy-related traits in predicting impersonal sex and hostile masculinity. Personality and Individual Differences. 2013 Oct;**55**(7):817-822

[92] Carton H, Egan V. The dark triad and intimate partner violence. Personality and Individual Differences. 2017;**105**:84-88

[93] Leedom LJ, Bass A, Almas LH. The problem of parental psychopathy. Journal of Child Custody. 2013;**10**(2):154-184

[94] Sociopaths and their Smear Campaigns. Lovefraudcom – Sociopaths Psychopaths Antisocials Con Artists Bigamists [Internet]. 2007. Available from: https://lovefraud.com/sociopaths-and-their-smear-campaigns/, https://plus.google.com/b/106129766857217075218/106129766857217075218/posts [Accessed: April 30, 2017]

[95] Gurman AS. A framework for the comparative study of couple therapy. In: Gurman AS, editor. Clinical Handbook of Couple Therapy. New York, NY, US: Guilford Press; 2008. pp. 1-26

[96] Oka M, Whiting JB. Contemporary MFT theories and intimate partner violence: A review of systemic treatments. Journal of Couple & Relationship Therapy. 2011;**10**(1):34-52

[97] Stowasser, J. E. EMDR and family therapy in the treatment of domestic violence. In F. Shapiro, F. W. Kaslow, & L. Maxfield (Eds.), Handbook of EMDR and family therapy processes. Hoboken, NJ: John Wiley & Sons Inc; 2007. p. 243-261

[98] DeBoer KM, Rowe LS, Frousakis NN, Dimidjian S, Christensen A. Couples excluded from a therapy trial due to intimate partner violence: Subsequent treatment-seeking and occurrence of IPV. Psychology of Violence. 2012;**2**(1):28

[99] Schacht RL, Dimidjian S, George WH, Berns SB. Domestic violence assessment procedures among couple therapists. Journal of Marital and Family Therapy. 2009;**35**(1):47-59

[100] Bograd M, Mederos F. Battering and couples therapy: Universal screening and selection of treatment modality. Journal of Marital and Family Therapy. 1999 Jul 1;**25**(3):291-312

[101] Leedom LJ, Andersen D, Glynn MA. Individual and couple therapy for intimate partner violence: Perpetrator personality disorder diagnosis and meaning making. Submitt Publ. 2017

[102] Leedom LJ. Just Like His Father? Fairfield, CT: Healing Arts Press; 2006

[103] Auty KM, Farrington DP, Coid JW. Intergenerational transmission of psychopathy and mediation via psychosocial risk factors. British Journal of Psychiatry. 2015;**206**(1):26-31

[104] Hare RD. Without Conscience: The Disturbing World of the Psychopaths Among Us. New York, NY, US: Guilford Press; 1999. p. 260

[105] Jaffee SR, Moffitt TE, Caspi A, Taylor A. Life with (or without) father: The benefits of living with two biological parents depend on the father's antisocial behavior. Child Development. 2003 Feb;**74**(1):109-126

[106] Moss HB, Lynch KG, Hardie TL, Baron DA. Family functioning and peer affiliation in children of fathers with antisocial personality disorder and substance dependence: Associations with problem behaviors. American Journal of Psychiatry. 2002 Apr;**159**(4):607-614

[107] Pfiffner LJ, McBurnett K, Rathouz PJ. Father absence and familial antisocial characteristics. Journal of Abnormal Child Psychology. 2001 Oct 1;**29**(5):357-367

[108] Kirkman CA. From soap opera to science: Towards gaining access to the psychopaths who live amongst us. Psychology and Psychotherapy. 2005 Sep;**78**(Pt 3):379-396

[109] Jaffee SR, Belsky J, Harrington H, Caspi A, Moffitt TE. When parents have a history of conduct disorder: How is the caregiving environment affected? Journal of Abnormal Psychology. 2006 May;**115**(2):309-319

[110] Blazei R, Iacono W, McGue M. Father-child transmission of antisocial behavior: The moderating role of father's presence in the home. Journal of the American Academy of Child & Adolescent Psychiatry. 2008 Apr;**47**(4):406-415

[111] DeGarmo DS. Coercive and prosocial fathering, antisocial personality, and growth in children's postdivorce noncompliance. Child Development. 2010 Mar;**81**(2):503-516

[112] Coley RL, Carrano J, Lewin-Bizan S. Unpacking links between fathers' antisocial behaviors and children's behavior problems: Direct, indirect, and interactive effects. Journal of Abnormal Child Psychology. 2011 Mar 1;**39**(6):791-804

[113] Thornberry TP, Freeman-Gallant A, Lovegrove PJ. Intergenerational linkages in antisocial behaviour. Criminal Behaviour and Mental Health. 2009;**19**(2):80-93

[114] Jacob T, Haber JR, Leonard KE, Rushe R. Home interactions of high and low antisocial male alcoholics and their families. Journal of Studies on Alcohol. 2000;**61**(1):72-80

[115] Febres J, Shorey RC, Zucosky HC, Brasfield H, Vitulano M, Elmquist J, et al. The relationship between male-perpetrated interparental aggression, paternal characteristics, and child psychosocial functioning. Journal of Child and Family Studies. 2013 Apr;**23**(5):907-916

[116] Bosquet M, Egeland B. Predicting parenting behaviors from antisocial practices content scale scores of the MMPI-2 administered during pregnancy. Journal of Personality Assessment. 2000 Feb;**74**(1):146-162

[117] Kim-Cohen J, Caspi A, Rutter M, Tomás MP, Moffitt TE. The caregiving environments provided to children by depressed mothers with or without an antisocial history. American Journal of Psychiatry. 2006 Jun;**163**(6):1009-1018

[118] Robinson BA, Azores-Gococo N, Brennan PA, Lilienfeld SO. The roles of maternal psychopathic traits, maternal antisocial personality traits, and parenting in the development of child psychopathic traits. Parenting, Science and Practice. 2016;**16**(1):36-55

[119] Loney BR, Huntenburg A, Counts-Allan C, Schmeelk KM. A preliminary examination of the intergenerational continuity of maternal psychopathic features. Aggressive Behavior. 2007;**33**(1):14-25

[120] Davies PT, Sturge-Apple ML, Cicchetti D, Manning LG, Vonhold SE. Pathways and processes of risk in associations among maternal antisocial personality symptoms, interparental aggression, and preschooler's psychology. Development and Psychopathology. 2012 Aug;**24**(3):807-832

[121] Sellers R, Harold GT, Elam K, Rhoades KA, Potter R, Mars B, et al. Maternal depression and co-occurring antisocial behaviour: Testing maternal hostility and warmth as mediators of risk for offspring psychopathology. Journal of Child Psychology and Psychiatry. 2014 Feb;**55**(2):112-120

[122] Ehrensaft MK, Wasserman GA, Verdelli L, Greenwald S, Miller LS, Davies M. Maternal antisocial behavior, parenting practices, and behavior problems in boys at risk for antisocial behavior. Journal of Child and Family Studies. 2003 Mar;**12**(1):27-40

[123] Beaver KM, da Silva Costa C, Poersch AP, Freddi MC, Stelmach MC, Connolly EJ, et al. Psychopathic personality traits and their influence on parenting quality: Results from a nationally representative sample of Americans. Psychiatric Quarterly. 2014 Dec;**85**(4):497-511

[124] Wilson S, Durbin CE. Parental personality disorder symptoms are associated with dysfunctional parent-child interactions during early childhood: A multilevel modeling analysis. Personality Disorders: Theory, Research, and Treatment. 2012;**3**(1):55

[125] Capaldi DM, Pears KC, Kerr DCR, Owen LD, Kim HK. Growth in externalizing and internalizing problems in childhood: A prospective study of psychopathology across three generations. Child Development. 2012 Nov;**83**(6):1945-1959

[126] Eaves LJ, Prom EC, Silberg JL. The mediating effect of parental neglect on adolescent and young adult anti-sociality: A longitudinal study of twins and their parents. Behavior Genetics. 2010 Jul;**40**(4):425-437

[127] Jouriles EN, Rosenfield D, McDonald R, Vu NL, Rancher C, Mueller V. Children exposed to intimate partner violence: Conduct problems, interventions, and partner contact with the child. Journal of Clinical Child & Adolescent Psychology. 2016 Jul;**1**:1-3

[128] McDonald R, Jouriles EN, Rosenfield D, Leahy MM. Children's questions about interparent conflict and violence: What's a mother to say? Journal of Family Psychology. 2012 Feb;**26**(1):95-104

[129] Johnson MP. Conflict and control gender symmetry and asymmetry in domestic violence. Violence Women. 2006;**12**(11):1003-1018

[130] Hannah MT. Domestic Violence, Abuse and Child Custody. Civic Research Institute; 2011. p. 704

[131] Baglivio MT, Jackowski K, Greenwald MA, Wolff KT. Comparison of multisystemic therapy and functional family therapy effectiveness: A multiyear statewide propensity score matching analysis of juvenile offenders. Criminal Justice and Behavior. 2014 Sep;**41**(9):1033-1056

[132] Rock RC, Sellbom M, Ben-Porath YS, Salekin RT. Concurrent and predictive validity of psychopathy in a batterers' intervention sample. Law and Human Behavior. 2013 Jun;**37**(3):145-154

[133] Andrews DA, Bonta J. The Psychology of Criminal Conduct [Internet]. 3rd ed. Cincinnati, OH, US: Anderson Publishing Co.; 2003. Available from: http://search.ebscohost.com/login.aspx?direct=true&db=psyh&AN=2005-11916-000&site=ehost-live

[134] Casey K. Evil Beside Her: The True Story of a Texas Woman's Marriage to a Dangerous Psychopath. HarperCollins; 2008. p. 389

Chapter 8

Psychopathy: The Reflection of Severe Psychosocial Dysfunction

Sevgi Güney

Additional information is available at the end of the chapter

http://dx.doi.org/10.5772/intechopen.72329

Abstract

Psychopathy is the result of the bundle of personality characteristics that typically displays socio-communicative impairment as well as restricted social skills and activities in which neurophysiological impairments are reported. The most prominent feature of psychopathy is that communication failures occur in interpersonal relations due to insincere charm for manipulations, grandiose self-perception, rule-breaking tendencies, irresponsibility and unpredictable impulsive behaviors. Since the individuals with psychopathic traits are very self-centered, they act on their emotional state. Their behaviors are driven by feelings and impulsive wishes. That is why, they are untrustable individuals. They have lots of difficulty and are considered to be dangerous in maintaining long-term relationships, particularly with their intimate partner. It is a critical mistake to assume that psychopathy is caused by the individual's incomplete individuality. This mistake leads to inability to be eliminated of the problems in not only correctional interventions in forensic settings but also treatment procedures in clinical settings. In this chapter, the characteristics of psychopathy are explained for providing some inspiration in the line of successful treatment procedures and intervention strategies in forensic and clinical settings.

Keywords: psychopathy, impairment, forensic clinical psychology, criminal psychology

1. Introduction

Psychopathy is a personality traits bundle, which is the reflection of organizational personality problems during childhood and adolescent period and a personality disorder in adulthood. They have suffered from a kind of inability to develop genuine relationships with teachers, friends, or people with intimate relationships.

The motivation of human behaviors in daily life are directed via feelings and thinking structures. Human behaviors, on the other hand, have been emerged in the direction of the thoughts combined with sentiments, making sense, abstraction and inference. Therefore, there should be "knowledge" that directly contributes to the formation of philosophies and emotions underlying the behavior. Where does "knowledge" come from? Moreover, it is accepted that emotions have evolved from the influence of external factors on the areas of the brain. The external factors include genes, family environment, social environment and psychosocial development periods. Collectively, these factors are effective in the formation of our thoughts and feelings that underlie our behavior that reveals our motivation too. Emotions contribute to the formation of behaviors via matching experiences. As evolutionary psychologists have pointed out, brain, central nervous system has established appropriate systems for protecting the individual from sudden situations that constitute a rapid change of feelings. These systems are in the form of the transferred patterns for generations. These systems come together and help to regulate our behaviors. The oxytocin is very effective in the activation of these systems. The experimental studies have pointed out that there is significant impairment in the release of oxytocin in the individuals with psychopathy.

2. The characteristics of the individuals with psychopathy

The individual with psychopathy has limited and also superficial affective processing with respect to remorse and anticipatory anxiety. Since impulsivity is one of the featured behavioral styles, general failure is inevitable to evaluate anticipated actions and to inhibit the inappropriate ones. As psychopathy is a bunch of personality characteristics rather than a disorder in itself, this perspective allows us to see the fact that psychopathy can also occur in other mental health disorders. Most professionals wrongly consider the psychopathic behavioral patterns as a sign of antisocial and sociopathic personality disorder. There is a huge amount of research studies suggesting that antisocial behaviors are the consequences of the emotional/affective impairments. This should not be taken into account as antisocial personality disorder. The individuals with psychopathy display focused aversive events and even "cold-blooded" criminal behaviors. The misunderstanding leads to misdescription of the psychopathic behavior pattern's etiology. The concept of psychopathy is negatively effective in human behavior so that it becomes an important phenomenon for behavioral modification studies, correctional works and also treatment procedure in clinical setting. This importance derives not only from the definition of the problem but also from the fact that the individual and social building blocks involved in the psychosocial development of the individual are negatively and occasionally destructive. Some professionals believe in behaviors on the axis of psychopathic thought content result of the individual's incomplete or misplaced individuality. This is an incomplete description. True, but incomplete! Psychopathy must be dealt with in the social context in which it interacts with the individual as the "knowledge" directly contributes to the formation of the philosophies underlying the behavior.

Numerous studies have been conducted to investigate the etiology of psychopathy [2–4, 19, 38]. After many studies, it is generally accepted that lack of emotion (this feature may makes them "cold-blooded" [62, 27, 28]) and remorse is the core feature of psychopathy, whereas there is still debate as to whether criminal behavior is a necessary feature of it or not [23]. Moreover, it has been suggested that antisocial behavior is the consequence of the affective impairments, which should not be considered as one of the diagnostic criteria [6–8].

It is good to redefine the question "what is psychopathy?" Some authors such as Cleckley called psychopathy as the mask of sanity [11]. Since 1941, Cleckley has been trying to conceptualize a psychopathic person's thinking styles. According to Cleckley's conceptualization, psychopathic individuals as a perfect copy of normally functioning individuals, able to mask their internal chaos being resulted in purposeful destructive behavior, often more self-destructive than destructive to others. Although intelligent, even charming external presentation has attracted attention, the individuals with psychopathy do not have the ability to experience genuine emotions internally. Cleckley investigates whether the mask of sanity is intentionally preferred to hide the lack of internal structure or the mask just results from semantic neuropsychological deficits. He concluded that it is an unidentified semantic impairment. It is claimed that there are 16 common defined criteria universally. These are lack of guilt, egocentricity, dishonesty, lack of anxiety, superficial charm, undependability, failure to learn from punishment, lack of insight into the impact of one's behavior on others, failure to plan ahead, lack of emotions and failure to form long-term intimate relationships. Thus, psychopathy consists of multiple components ranging from the emotional, cognitive, interpersonal and behavioral spectrum. To catch the problem, both evidence-based and also at an early stage, objective measurement devices were developed. Psychopathy Checklist-Revised [24] is one of the most effective scientific measures among them. In many judicial institutions, it is part of best practiced protocols as it is well-designed to measure the psychopathic traits such as antisocial traits, behaviors, lifestyle, interpersonal and affective impairments. The individuals with psychopathy in their interpersonal relationships present grandiose, deceptive, dominant, manipulative, superficial, unable to form strong emotional bonds with others, affectively shallow, irresponsible, impulsive, tend to ignore social conventions, lacking in empathy, guilt and/or remorse characteristics [33].

3. The neural explanations on psychopathy

The ability of psychopathic individuals to empathize with others' feelings is quite different than normal individuals. The individuals with psychopathic traits have limited arousal to the emotions of others [37, 39]. Dealing with their affective functioning, while they are watching videos depicting expression of pain, it is expected that higher activity in brain areas is involved in the affective response such as amygdala, the insula, as well as higher subjective ratings of personal distress [43]. However, individuals with psychopathic traits show less response than healthy ones. Neuroimaging studies examine the relevant brain regions and circuits being implicated in the condition of the orbitofrontal cortex, amygdala, and the anterior and posterior cingulate and adjacent (para)limbic structures of individuals with psychopathy. It is accepted that there is somehow a prefrontal lobe structure deficit in them [3, 20]. Perhaps, due to this deficit, the low arousal, poor fear conditioning, lack of conscience and decision-making deficits have characterized the psychopathic actions [52]. Lockwood et al. [36] in their study examined the neural response of children with conduct problems by using functional magnetic resonance imaging (fMRI). They measured the neural responses to the pictures of others in pain with a large sample of children with conduct problems. They found that these children displayed atypical empathic responses and callous traits to others, and also conferred some risk for adult psychopathy. These children showed reduced blood oxygen level-dependent responses to others' pain in bilateral anterior insula, anterior cingulate cortex and inferior frontal gyrus, regions related with empathy for pain.

There is a series of models having attempted to account for the neurological functional impairments existed by the individuals with psychopathy. These are the left hemisphere activation hypothesis, the various positions proposing frontal lobe dysfunction, and finally, the somatic marker [14–16, 40, 49, 50, 52].

3.1. The left hemisphere activation hypothesis model

According to the model, individuals with psychopathy have been suffered from unusual lateralization of language function. They may have fewer left hemisphere resources for processing language than the normal ones [25, 9]. Hare have found that individuals with psychopathy showed pronounced difficulty for the abstract category discrimination [24]. If the stimuli were presented at the left visual field, it is still unclear to what degree they are. There is a lack of specificity about why greater activation of left hemisphere systems disrupts the cortical functioning. There are some indicators of the "unusual" lateralization of language function in individuals with psychopathy. Unfortunately, there are no clear reasons why these impairments give rise to the development of psychopathy. All data from the experimental studies have been indicated that the excessive activation of the left hemisphere somehow has effect on cognitive processing but the direction and which conditions lead to this, is still unclear.

3.2. The frontal lobe dysfunction hypothesis model

The authors claimed that psychopathic traits may occur due to frontal lobe dysfunctions [44, 40, 43]. This hypothesis was derived from three sets of data of patients with acquired lesions of frontal cortex, the neuropsychological studies on the individuals with antisocial traits and the neuroimaging studies on the individuals with antisocial behaviors. There is a common knowledge about frontal lobe dysfunction that it increases the risk of aggressive behavior. The patients with orbital and medial frontal cortex lesions are more likely to act in aggressive manner. It is known that aggressive individuals display impaired performance, impaired executive functions and present with reduced frontal activity during rest conditions [20]. However, the frontal lobe dysfunctional positions remain still unspecified. The experimental studies do not distinguish between different regions of prefrontal cortex, different forms of executive functions, and/or at the behavioral level, between reactive and instrumental aggression. The model, moreover, have failed to provide any detailed cognitive explanation as to why damaged functions mediated by frontal cortex lead to an increased risk of aggression [14].

3.3. The somatic marker hypothesis model

The somatic markers of this healthy individual provide affective coloring being automatically bias toward behaviors or a way from the available response options. In other words, the somatic marker provides an automated way of labeling a particular response being made. The rapid labeling occurs via "body loop" in which a "somatic marker" is conveyed to somatosensory cortices but it can also occur via an "as-if body loop" in which the body is by passed and reactivation signals are conveyed to the somatosensory structures. The somatosensory pattern marks the scenario as either good or bad, allowing the rapid reflection [15, 22]. Individuals with psychopathy appear to generate impaired somatic markers. Especially dealing with reactive aggression, the acting mechanism may occur in the manner of "hit that person but be punished later." In a healthy individual, there will be activation of the linkage between knowledge of hitting and punishment and the emotional aversion to punishment. The consequent aversive somatic marker guides the healthy individual away from hitting the other. However, the individuals with psychopathy have suffered from the impairment in the somatic marker system. Thus, there is no somatic marker to guide their behavior. Therefore, it can be expected a similar outcome for instrumental aggression in these individuals.

Generally, dealing with neural explanations of psychopathy, there are both clear and unproven conclusions. It is clear that frontal lobe dysfunction may lead to increase in aggression. The dorsolateral executive dysfunction may be related to reactive antisocial behavior, but the relation is only correlational not causal. In contrast, ventral-medial and orbital frontal cortex dysfunction are causally associated with a heightened risk of reactive aggression. Dealing with the psychopathic acts, there are reasons to consider the maladaptive behaviors in psychopathy may be related to orbital and medial cortex dysfunctions. To what extent, these dysfunctions are causal is not clear enough. Much of work should be done to explain why frontal lesions increase the probability of reactive aggression and also psychopathic acts. In this regard, the somatic markers hypothesis can be taken into account, but the hypothesis has not had adequate scientifically proven explanations for reactive and instrumental aggression.

4. The cognitive explanations on psychopathy

As human behaviors directed by information processing strategies, here the term cognitive refers to information processing [9]. Thus, there are three main information processing models in the line of explaining the cognitive components of psychopathic thinking styles and behaviors [63]. These are the response set modulation hypothesis, Newman [43], the fear dysfunction models [19, 5, 38] violence inhibition mechanism model, Blair (1995), left hemisphere activation hypothesis, Kosson (1996), Frontal lobe dysfunction model, [22, 50, 51] and the Somatic Marker Hypothesis, Damasio (1994). The last three models focus primarily on the neural structure and level of the pattern. To provide a brief overview on the etiology of the psychopathy, these models will be described shortly.

4.1. The response set modulation model

The model pointed out "a rapid and relatively automatic shift of attention from the effortful organization and implementation of goal-directed behavior to its evaluation" [43]. This brief and highly automatic shift of attention enables the individual to monitor and use information being peripheral to their dominant response set (i.e., "deliberate focus of attention" [37]. The physiological explanation of the model was based on the theory of Gray's Septo-Hippocampal Lesions for Emotional Learning [44]. We know the individual with psychopathy has reduced automatic processing. Newman has explained this as "whereas most people automatically anticipate the consequences of their actions, automatically feel shame for unkind deeds, automatically understand why they should persist in the face of frustration, automatically distrust propositions that seem too good to be true and are automatically aware of their commitments to others, psychopaths may only become aware of such factors with effort". Shortly according to the Newman's model, individuals with psychopathy are not incapable of regulating his/her behaviors, they only need much more effort to regulate their behavior as there is a lack of "normal people automatic information processing" to guide their actions. The remarkable psychopathic characteristics such as impulsivity, poor passive avoidance and emotion-processing deficits can be dealt with a failure to process the meaning of information being perhaps incidental to their deliberate focus of attention [38]. Their actions called as goal-directed activity and in some circumstances as top-down directed attention process. Top-down attention modulates amygdala activation especially in psychopathy. For a long time, it is attributed that psychopathic acts are a fundamental deficit in fear arising from impaired amygdala function (Larson et al., 2013). The response set modulation model is an attention-based model. Individuals with psychopathy always operate under high load conditions during their goal-directed activities and/or top-down directed attention process. Their both goal-directed activities and top-down directed attention process are very effective so that they fail to incorporate other stimulus dimensions. In other words, attention to target stimuli dimensions so suppresses the representation of the unattended stimuli being not processed.

4.2. The dysfunctional fear hypothesis model

This model defends the fact that there is impairment in the neurophysiological systems modulating fear behavior in individuals with psychopathy. They appear almost as incapable of profound remorse ([11], p. 340). Their moral socialization process is completed through the suffering from the use of punishment [19]. A healthy individual is frightened by punishment and decide not to engage in the actions causing punishment in the future. However, in psychopathic individuals, the fear-associated startle reflex has been found to be diminished or absent [46, 48]. The studies suggested that somehow there is a deficit in the amygdala in psychopathic individuals. Moreover, the imaging studies conducted recently have revealed a reduced activity in limbic circuits including amygdala in the individuals with psychopathy. Research on functional and structural frontal brain abnormalities has pointed out the evidence of decreased activity in orbito-frontal and limbic regions [4] and reduced prefrontal volume of gray matter [4, 50, 53, 65].

4.3. Violence inhibition mechanism (VIM) model

The model had been meant to detail a cognitive model of the prerequisites for human moral socialization. Moral socialization occurs through the pairing of the mechanism by distress cues with representations of the acts causing the distress cues [61]. By association, these representations become triggers for the mechanism. The child from "normal development period" initially finds the pain of other individuals aversive and then through socialization, thoughts of acts that cause pain to others become aversive. It has been suggested that individuals with psychopathy have disruption to this system such that representations of acts causing harm to others do not become triggers for the violence inhibition mechanism model [61] (Blair et al. 2001b, Steven et al., 2001). Although the VIM model provides an explanation on the emergence of the instrumental antisocial behavior displayed by the individuals with psychopathy, it cannot account for the range of impairments shown by the individuals. The model cannot give reasonable explanation dealing with the response set modulation and fear hypotheses. This shortage leads to an expansion of the model at both cognitive and neural levels which is called "the integrated emotion systems model." Finally, none of these three cognitive models can provide an adequate explanation of psychopathy. By the way, contrary to social and psychodynamic theories, these three models provide significant scientific tips not only for psycho-bio-social theories but also for neuropsychological research studies at least.

5. Crime and psychopathy

Crime is an act fulfilled by social, psychological and biological factors. No one can say that criminal behavior is caused only by social factors. As everyone knows, social causes of crime have also psychological pathways. Individuals behave differently in their psychosocial conditions in the face of unlawful life events. The personality and intelligence of all human beings concerned filter objective conditions and determine their perception. For example, poverty may cause some people to rebel against the authority—government and even a society, while others blame themselves, their lack of cognitive ability, their ignorance and perhaps on their incapable skills. These factors are well-documented by the authors such as Lazarus [13].

To understand the relation between a criminal behavior and psychopathy, we should try to understand the causal pathways involved. Recidivism is another important concept as the concept corresponds to an act of an individual repeating a criminal behavior, a habitual relapse and a chronic tendency toward repetition of the criminal acts [44, 47, 30]. In this regard, we come to mention of the "personality dimensions" [46, 48]. Why do most of us act in a socially desirable way, while some others do not? In fact criminals know what is right and wrong except the mentally retarded criminals. They just prefer "the wrong" to the right. Why? The literature pointed out roughly three conditions":

1. Individuals who do not have enough socially approved experiences. In other words, parents, teachers and even peers cannot give a child proper reinforcers.

2. Somehow, the wrong experiences are reinforced. Even in some local cultures, parents encourage their children to act aggressively and in an inappropriate way. The parents prefer to use much more punishment than reward to prepare their children for the hard and aversive life conditions [47].

3. Not being aware of the consequences of behaviors, but repeating those behaviors over and over.

Since individuals with psychopathy do not have knowledge of the consequences of their actions, they do not realize that all the disturbing life events they experience are just because of their actions and thinking styles, in short being themselves [42].

It is obvious that social causes of crime have psychological pathways. Every individual acts differently to inequality, poverty and injustice. These all may lead to some individuals to act unlawfully against society while others blame themselves, their ignorance, their lack of skill and even they perceive unemployment as just punishment to themselves [32, 33]. As mental health professionals, we know that the nature of some personality traits such as psychopathy is quite related to criminal behaviors. The chain begins with DNA, since DNA is the genetic structure underlying individual differences. The evidence from literature shows clearly that most of the variance for individual differences in personality is due to both genetic causes [64, 65] and social environment where the individual has been born and grown in [54, 57, 58]. These two sources of individual differences constitute the distal and proximal antecedent conditions for individual differences.

No doubt, there are no genes for criminality but there is a risk of criminal behavior through the genes coding for structural proteins and enzymes influencing metabolic, hormonal and the other physiological processes [62, 63]. Why do most of people not act in criminal behavior? It is because of the laws. By the way, some people have a strong tendency to be "a criminal." Do those people not know about the laws? No, they know as well as anybody. However they prefer to act as the wrong to the right. When we react to something, if it is wrong we are punished by our parents, our teachers, our peers, and so on, but when we act in a socially approved way, we are rewarded. Every occasion serves to reinforce how we act. These experiences are conditioned and are called as "conscience." There is a lot of evidence that psychopathic individuals and criminals show relatively poor conditionability compared with "normal" individuals [24, 29, 41]. Raine claims that arousal has effects on criminality [51–53]. The criminals have psychopathic personality characteristics and acts [42, 31]. Research shows that there is converging evidence for the powerful relation between psychopathy and serious repetitive crime, violent behavior, instrumental and "cold-blooded" violence and violent behavior [38, 25, 10]. What can be done? How can it be reduced? Increasing severity of punishment would not have a large positive effect. As we know that trouble behaviors in kindergarten are relatively predictive of later criminal act, deviant behaviors and psychopathic tendencies. It is adequate to conduct longitudinal training programs and prevention programs as much as earlier stages of the developmental process. It is well-known that one caution should be given on the occasion of the first offense, but serious punishment should follow the next offense. Moreover, nowadays, we know that correctional interventions must be based on behavioral approaches taking root from learning theories. Psychologists also suggest that correlations of future criminality can be found in early childhood. What does it mean? It means that the prevention programs must began with early childhood educational systems. School, certainly, has deeply a civilizing influence. Finally, it is so important to educate the parents in the line to teach their children to exist themselves without entering into the personal sphere of the others. The child growing up with the awareness of the personal sphere learns to respect the rights of others.

6. Psychopathy and other mental disorders

In classification systems, psychopathy appears in childhood, adolescent and adulthood disorders. In childhood and adolescent period, it emerges as a conduct disorder before the age of 15 and antisocial personality disorder as in the adulthood. The psychopathic characteristics include aggressive and destructive behaviors on one side and deceitfulness and/or theft, non-aggressive rule-breaking behaviors on the other side [34, 35, 39].

Repeated illegal acts, impulsiveness, hostile-aggressive behavior, acts endangering self or others, failure to make stable future plans and deceitfulness are the most common features of an individual with psychopathic traits in adulthood. The age criterion is at least 18 years old.

Psychopathy in childhood is manifested as conduct disorder [59]. It is apparent as aggression toward people or animals, destruction of property, deceptiveness or stealing and serious rule violations. Achenbach [1] created Child Behavior Checklist to define aggressive and delinquent behavior syndrome in childhood.

It is accepted that individuals with psychopathy often are violent [26]. They can use all of our empathy against us. Schizophrenics tend to live in an uncertain world being malevolent. Actually, schizophrenia is a heartbreaking disease. A schizophrenic may hear, see and believe things that are simply not real. This of course depends also on their psychotic level. It is known that schizophrenia is a psychotic disorder prominented by highly severe impaired thinking, emotions and behaviors. Patients with schizophrenia typically cannot filter sensory stimuli and may have impaired perceptions of sounds, colors and other factors of their environment [45, 60]. Most of them gradually withdraw from their social interactions and also lose ability to engage their personal hygiene and needs.

Bipolar patients may act as psychopath. The patients especially in manic episode may display psychopathic behavioral patterns. In this period, they may be callous. As grandiose thinking style is at the forefront, they may act in the form of rule breaking, have a strong tendency for criminality but all these may only occur in the manic episode and are curable. Individuals with psychopathy permanently have all of these vulnerabilities.

Borderline disorder may include some psychopathic tendencies. They sometimes behave like individuals with psychopathy. They have basic trust issues and also needy and demanding characteristics. Borderline individuals cannot be "goal directed." In contrast with borderline patients, individuals with psychopathy is self-assured, has appropriate plan for manipulation of the others and they can easily continue with their plans, and "cold-blooded." Individuals with psychopathy never have a history of suicidal acts, they engage in acts such as calculated controlling and manipulation of the others.

There have been a few studies searching at the comorbid psychopathy in schizophrenic patients. Violent patients with schizophrenia have higher psychopathy scores than those who are not violent [45]. These patients also have a higher number of criminal acts [56, 60]. Some authors claim that psychopathy is a robust predictor of violent, recidivism especially in patients with schizophrenia [61, 55]. On the other hand, there is no study that includes more detailed dimensional measures of personality and interpersonal relations of the patient population.

Dealing with the connection between schizophrenia and psychopathy could be more criminal. The patients have higher trait impulsivity and aggression scores on psychometric assessments [17, 18]. They have less self-control, more aggressive, deviant and impulsive personality style [12, 21].

People with psychosis have lost the capacity to think and behave rationally. This impairment results in breaking the bond with reality. The patient become bizarre and begins to have delusions, experience false perceptions such as hallucinations. Individuals with psychopathy may be in psychotic state as a result of many different underlying conditions; sometimes brain tumors and/or some of physical abnormalities. This is called pseudo psychosis as when the appropriate medical treatment is applied, psychotic symptoms disappear. Moreover, Alzheimer's and other types of dementia also cause a kind of psychotic state.

Author details

Sevgi Güney

Address all correspondence to: sevgiguney@gmail.com

Ankara University, Ankara, Turkey

References

[1] Achenbach TM. Manual Fort he Child Behavior Checklist/4-18, Burlington (Vermont) University of Vermont. VIT, USA: Department of Psychiatry; 1991

[2] Adolphs A, Tranel D, Damasio H, Damasio A. Impaired recognition of emotion in facial expressions following bilateral damage to the human amigdala. Nature. 1994;**372**:669-672

[3] Anderson NE, Kiehl KA. The psychopath magnetized: Insights from brain imaging. Trends in Cognitive Sciences. 2012;**16**:52-60

[4] Baskin-Sommers AR, Neumann CS, Cope L, Kiehl KA. Latent variable modeling of brain gray matter volume and psychopathy in incarcerated offenders. Journal of Abnormal Psychology. 2016;**125**:811-817. DOI: 10.1037/abn0000175

[5] Birbaumer N, Veit R, Lotze M, Erb M, Hermann C, Grodd W, Flor H. Deficient fear conditioning in psychopathy: A functional magnetic resonance imaging study. Archives of General Psychiatry. 2005;**62**:799-805

[6] Blair RJ, Mitchell DG. Psychopathy, attention and emotion. Psychological Medicine. 2009;**39**:543-555

[7] Blair RJ. Responding to the emotions of others: Dissociating forms of empathy through the study of typical and psychiatric populations. Consciousness and Cognition. 2005;**14**:698-718. DOI: 10.1016/j.concog.2005.06.004

[8] Briken P, Hill A, Berner W. Pharmacotherapy of paraphilias with long-acting agonists of luteinizing hormone-releasing hormone: A systematic review. Journal of Clinical Psychiatry. 2003;**64**:890-897

[9] Brook M, Kosson DS. Impaired cognitive empathy in criminal psychopathy: Evidence from a laboratory measure of empathic accuracy. Journal of Abnormal Psychology. 2013;156-166. DOI: 10.1037/a0030261

[10] Brown AR, Dargis MA, Mattern AC, Tsonis MA, Newman JP. Elevated psychopathy scores among mixed sexual offender: Replication and extension. Criminal Justice and Behavior. 2015;**42**:1032-1044. DOI: 10.1177/0093854815575389

[11] Cleckley HM. The mask of sanity. 5th ed. St. Louis, MO: Mosby; 2015

[12] Coffley M, Coleman M. The relationship between support and stress in forensic community mental health nursing. Journal of Advances in. Nursing. 2001;**34**:397-407

[13] Daversa MT. Early environment predictors of the affective and interpersonal constructs of psychopathy. International Journal of Offender Therapy and Comparative Criminology. 2010;**54**(1):6-21. DOI: 10.1177/0306624X08328754

[14] Decety J, Chenyi C, Harenski C, Kiehl KA. Neurological basis for lack of empathy in psychopaths. Frontiers in Human Neuroscience. 2013;**7**:489. DOI: 10.3389/fnhum.2013.00489

[15] Decety J, Skelly L, Yoder KJ, Kiehl KA. Neural processing of dynamic emotional facial expressions in psychopaths. Social Neuroscience. 2014;**9**(1):36-49. DOI: 10.1080/17470919.2013.866905

[16] Dolan M. Psychopathy—A neurobiological perspective. British Journal of Psychiatry. 1994;**165**:151-159

[17] Dolan M, Blackburn M. Interpersonal factors as predictors of disciplinary infractions in incarcerated personality disordered offenders. Personality and Individual Differences. 2006;**40**:897-907

[18] Edens JF, Marcus DK, Lilienfeld SO, Poythress NG. Psychopathic, not psychopath: Taxometric evidence for the dimensional structure of psychopathy. Journal of Abnormal Psychology. 2006;**115**:131-144

[19] Eysenck M, Gudjonhsson GH. The Causes and Cures of Criminality. Boston, MA: Springer; 1989. DOI: https://doi.org/10.1007/978-1-4757-6726-1

[20] Fecteau S, Pascual-Leone A, Theoret H. Psychopathy and the mirror neuron system: Preliminary findings from a non-psychiatric sample. Psychiatry Research. 2008;**160**: 137144. DOI: 10.1016/j.psychres.2007.08.022

[21] Fullam R, Dolan M. The criminal and personality profile of patients with schizophrenia and comorbid psychopathic traits. Personality and Individual Differences. 2006;**40**:1591-1602

[22] Glenn AL, Raine A. Psychopathy: An introduction to biological findings and their implications. New York, NY: NYU Press; 2014

[23] Hall JR, Benning SD. The "successful" psychopath: Adaptive and subclinical manifestations of psychopathy in the general population. In: Patrick CJ, editor. Handbook of Psychopathy. New York, NY: Guildford Press; 2006

[24] Hare RD. Psychopathy, the PCL-R, and criminal justice: Some new findings and current issues. Canadian Psychology. 2016;**57**:21-34. DOI: 10.1037/cap0000041

[25] Hare RD, Jutai JW. Psychopathy and cerebral asymmetry in semantic processing. Personality and Individual Differences. 1988;**9**(2):329-337. DOI: 10.1016/0191-8869(88)90095-5

[26] Harris GT, Rice ME. Treatment of psychopathy: A review of empirical findings. In: Patrick CJ, editor. Handbook of Psychopathy. New York: Guilford Press; 2006. pp. 555-572

[27] Herpertz SC, Sass H. Emotional deficiency and psychopathy. Behavioral Sciences & the Law. 2000;**18**:567-580

[28] Hodgins S, Hiscoke UL, Freese R. The antecedent of aggressive behavior among men with schizophrenia: A prospective investigation of patients in community treatment. Behavioural Sciences and the Law. 2003;**21**:523-546

[29] Kastner RM, Sellbom M. Hypersexuality in college students: The role of psychopathy. Personality and Individual Differences. 2012;**53**:644-649. DOI: 10.1016/j.paid.2012.05.005

[30] Kim SW, Grant JE. An open naltrexone treatment study in pathological gambling disorder. International Clinical Psychopharmacology. 2001;**16**:285-289

[31] Krstic S, Knight RA, Robertson CA. Developmental antecedents of the facets of psychopathy: The role of multiple abuse experiences. Journal of Personality Disorders. 2016;**29**:117. DOI: 10.1521/pedi_2015_29_223

[32] Krstic S, Neumann CS, Roy S, Robertson C, Knight RA, Hare RD. Using latent variable- and person-centered approaches to examine the role of psychopathic traits in sex offenders. Personality Disorders: Theory, Research, and Treatment. 2017. DOI: 10.1037/per0000249

[33] Krueger RF, Hicks B, Patrick CJ, Carlson S, Iacono WG, McGue M. Etiologic connections among substance dependence, antisocial behavior and personality: Modeling the externalizing spectrum. Journal of Abnormal Psychology. 2002;**111**:411-424

[34] Krueger RF. Personality traits in late adolescence predict mental disorders in early adulthood: A prospective—Epidemiological study. Journal of Personality. 1999;**67**:39-65

[35] Krueger RF, Markon KE, Patrick CJ, Iacono WG. Externalizing psychopathology in adulthood: A dimensional—Spectrum conceptualization and its implications for DSMV. Journal of Abnormal Psychology. 2005;**114**:537-550

[36] Lockwood PL, Sebastian CL, McCrory EJ, Hyde ZH, Gu X, De Brito SA, et al. Association of callous traits with reduced neural response to others' pain in children with conduct problems. Current Biology. 2013;**23**:1-5. DOI: 10.1016/j.cub.2013.04.018

[37] Lorenz AR, Newman JP. Do emotion and information processing deficiencies found in Caucasian psychopaths generalize to African–American psychopaths? Personality and Individual Differences. 2002;**32**:1077-1086

[38] Lykken DT. Psychopathy personality: The scope of the problem. In: Patrick CJ, editor. Handbook of Psychopathy. New York, NY: Guilford Press; 2007. pp. 3-13

[39] Minzenberg MJ, Siever L. Neurochemistry and pharmacology of psychopathy and related disorders. In: Patrick CJ, editor. Handbook of Psychopathy. New York: Guilford Press; 2006. pp. 251-277

[40] Moffitt TE. The neuropsychology of conduct disorder. Development and Psychopathology. 1993;**5**:135-151

[41] Mokros A, Hare RD, Neumann CS, Santtila P, Habermeyer E, Nitschke J. Variants of psychopathy in adult male offenders: A latent profile analysis. Journal of Abnormal Psychology. 2015;**124**:372-386. DOI: 10.1037/abn0000042

[42] Neumann CS, Hare RD, Pardini DA. Antisociality and the construct of psychopathy: Data from across the globe. Journal of Personality. 2015;**83**:678-692. DOI: 10.1111/jopy.12127

[43] Newman JP, Schmitt WA, Voss WS. The impact of motivationally neutral cues on psychopathic individuals: Assessing the generality of the response modulation hypothesis. Journal of Abnormal Psychology. 1997;**106**:563-575

[44] Newman JP, Curtin JJ, Bertsch JD, Baskin-Sommers AR. Attention moderates the fearlessness of psychopathic offenders. Biological Psychiatry. 2010;**67**:66-70

[45] Nolan KA, Volavka J, Mohr P, Czobor P. Psychopathy and violent behavior among patients with schizophrenia or schizoaffective disorder. Psychiatric Services. 1999;**50**: 787-792

[46] Patrick CJ, Bradley MM, Lang PJ. Emotion in the criminal psychopath: Startle reflex modulation. Journal of Abnormal Psychology. 1993;**102**:82-92

[47] Patrick CJ, Cuthbert BN, Lang PJ. Emotion in the criminal psychopath: Fear image processing. Journal of Abnormal Psychology. 1994;**103**:523-534

[48] Patrick CJ. Emotion and psychopathy: Startling new insights. Psychophysiology. 1994;**31**:319-330

[49] Raine A. Schizotypal and borderline features in psychopathic criminals. Personality and Individual Differences. 1992;**13**:717-722

[50] Raine A. From genes to brain to antisocial behavior. Current Directions in Psychological Science. 2008;**17**(5):323-328

[51] Raine A, Buchsbaum M, LaCasse L. Brain abnormalities in murderers indicated by positron emission tomography. Biological Psychiatry. 1997;**42**:495-508

[52] Raine A. Antisocial behavior and psychophysiology: A biosocial perspective and a prefrontal dysfunction hypothesis. In: Stoff DM, Breiling J, Maser JD, editors. Handbook of Antisocial Behavior. New York: Wiley; 1997. pp. 289-303

[53] Raine A, Lencz T, Bihrle S, LaCasse L, Colletti P. Reduced prefrontal gray matter volume and reduced autonomic activity in antisocial personality disorder. Archives of General Psychiatry. 2000;**57**:119-127

[54] Ramanathan S, Balasubramanian N, Krishnadas R. Macroeconomic environment during infancy as a possible risk factor for adolescent behavioral problems. JAMA Psychiatry. 2013;**70**:218-225

[55] Rasmussen K, Levander S, Sletvold H. Aggressive and non aggressive schizophrenics: Symptom profile and neuropsychological differences. Psychology, Crime and Law. 1995;**2**:119-129

[56] Serin RC. Treatment responsivity in criminal psychopaths. Forum on Corrections Research. 1995;**7**(3):23-26

[57] Seto MC, Quinsey VL. Toward the future: Translating basic research into prevention and treatment strategies. In: Patrick CJ, editor. Handbook of Psychopathy. New York; 2006. pp. 589-601

[58] Sullivan EA, Kosson DS. Ethnic and cultural variations in psychopathy. In: Patrick CJ, editor. Handbook of Psychopathy. New York: Guilford Press; 2006. pp. 437-458

[59] Tackett JL, Krueger RF, Sawyer MG, Graetz BW. Subfactors of DSM-IV conduct disorder: Evidence and connections with syndromes from the child behavior checklist. Journal of Abnormal Child Psychology. 2003;**31**:647-654

[60] Tengström A, Hodgins S, Grann M, Langström N, Kullgren G. Schizophrenia and criminal offending: The role of psychopathy and substance use disorders. Criminal Justice and Behavior. 2004;**31**:367-391

[61] Tengström A, Grann M, Langström N, Kullgren G. Psychopathy (PCL-R) as a predictor of violent recidivism among criminal offenders with schizophrenia. Law and Human. Behaviour. 2000;**24**:45-58

[62] Welker KM, Lozoya E, Campbell JA, Neumann CS, Carré JM. Testosterone, cortisol, and psychopathic traits in men and women. Physiology & Behavior. 2014;**129**:230-236. DOI: 10.1016/j.physbeh.2014.02.057

[63] Woodworth M, Porter S. In cold blood: Characteristics of criminal homicides as a function of psychopathy. Journal of Abnormal Psychology. 2002;**111**:436-445

[64] Vukasovic T, Bratko D. Heritability of personality: A meta-analysis of behavior genetic studies. Psychological Bulletin. 2015;**141**:769-785

[65] Yang Y, Raine A, Lencz T, Bihrle S, LaCasse L, Colletti P. Volume reduction in prefrontal gray matter in unsuccessful criminal psychopaths. Biological Psychiatry. 2005;**57**:1103-1108

Chapter 9

Successful Psychopaths: A Contemporary Phenomenon

Floriana Irtelli and Enrico Vincenti

Additional information is available at the end of the chapter

http://dx.doi.org/10.5772/intechopen.70731

Abstract

The majority of empirical research on psychopathy involves forensic populations; however, researchers have recently turned their attention to the nature and implications of psychopathic features in the workplace, hence shedding light on the notion of "workplace psychopaths." Nowadays, many studies deal with successful people having a psychopathic outlook in a work environment. This is a contemporary phenomenon, originated during the 1990s. In this period, changing nature of work and business has created a general state of confusion due to increasing instability and competitiveness. In this social context, psychopathic personality aspects, such as the appearance of calm, confidence and other psychopathic tendencies, are mistaken for "leadership qualities." This contemporary phenomenon is dangerous and connected to psychosocial risks: the social and environmental contexts are affected by this dynamic, which can for instance lead to increasing anxiety in the co-workers and lack of motivation. This affects not only workers, but also companies: results of recent researches show the significant influence of psychopaths on organizational commitment. These dynamics stimulated the interest of researchers in a variety of disciplines: psychiatry, as well as psychology, criminology, and sociology. This chapter aims at reviewing the current knowledge on this phenomenon, and to promote prevention and diagnosis.

Keywords: review, prevention, corporate psychopathy, antisocial, toxic leaders, business, contemporary phenomenon, psychopathic personality, snakes in suits, workplace psychopaths, executive psychopaths, industrial psychopaths, organizational psychopaths

1. Introduction

Corporate psychopathy is a new emerging concept, therefore the literature about this topic is relatively limited [1] this is why there is the need for a growing research on it. Specifically the concept of "corporate psychopath" represent the merging of the term "corporate," which relates to the business world, with the term "psychopath," which is typical of the psychological literature, to denote a person with a psychopathic personality who is active (often times undisturbed) in the organizational area [2]. Corporate psychopaths are subclinical psychopaths within a workplace; as a matter of fact it is necessary to specify that, while psychopaths are over-represented in the prison population, many psychopathic persons are non-violent members of the community [3, 4]. In the 1960s, psychosocial research in the work environment highlighted the impact of some aspects of the workplace on health [5], but in particular during the 1990s, changing nature of business in times of economic uncertainty, has created a general state of confusion, due to increasing instability and competitiveness: the 1990s change became a matter of business necessity and economic survival [6, 7]. In the period of "casino capitalism" [8] managers are reported to be experiencing circumstances like increasing intense work pressures [9, 10], very fast turnover of personnel, the growing problem of time pressure across modern society, increasing pace of business, and relatively shallow appointment procedures [10, 11], which often do not uncover some of their personality flaws [10, 12]. Today it is also essential for companies to maintain high productivity levels, despite the decreasing of economic resources [13] and the proliferation of time constraints, which can often have a brutalizing effect by leading managers to allocate insufficient time for empathic interaction with others: these aspects may have caused vicious cycles between culture individuals and society; in fact some theories have attempted to explain how modern business has facilitated the rise of psychopathic managers, which has in turn influenced capitalism [10, 12, 14, 15]. Research has suggested that psychopathy can even confer benefit on persons seeking rewards within a corporate setting [16], which indicates they can rise to the top of corporations [3, 17] coherently they have also been named as corporate psychopaths, industrial psychopaths, executive psychopaths, to differentiate them from their more commonly known criminal peers [10, 18–22]. Research has also suggested that business has promoted psychopathic managers because of their ruthless willingness to "get the job done," and as they attain senior positions, executive psychopaths have become architects of ruthlessness as they create a "culture of extremes" [10] so corporate psychopathy flourishes perhaps as the most significant threat to ethical corporate behavior. In this contemporary social context, psychopathic personality aspects, like the appearance of confidence, calm, strength, and other psychopathic dispositions, such as the disinclination to express emotions (except to manipulate), are often mistaken for "leadership qualities" [23], also because it is believed that the ability to remain calm and unemotional in pressured circumstances may be factors of success in business [10, 24, 25]. Their characteristics of being ultra-rational financially-oriented managers, with no emotional concern for or empathy with other employees [26], marks them appear as well-sitting in capitalistic context [27] that is profit oriented [10]. The psychopathic individuals' lack of caring allows them to use any means to achieve their objectives, thereby potentially causing harm to others. Psychopaths have in fact ever-worsening behaviors at a greater pace as they attempt to achieve their goals before anyone else. Psychopathy in these aspects has not necessarily been (superficially) considered an impediment to global corporate advancement because aspects like risk taking, low fear, and lack of concern for consequences are popularly associated with strong leadership styles and ambition [3, 28]. These attitudes are added to their conscience-free approach to life and willingness to lie to present themselves in the best possible light. Using the "mask of sanity" [3], psychopaths are "social chameleons" [29] and adjust their personality depending on the person they are interacting with [6, 7]. Despite these aspects, organizational psychopaths are frequently seen as being charming "organizational stars" deserving of awards by those above them (while they subject those below them to intimidation, bullying, and coercion). Actually successful psychopaths are assumed to have the potential to transform a company's organizational culture at their pleasing, which others must follow or else exit the company [7, 30], in fact through their attractive interpersonal communication styles, these subclinical psychopaths can influence others by becoming the "leader" [30], and particular significance is the personality of a/the top manager, since his/her personality will most greatly impact the managerial culture [1]. This poses an important ethical problem because it is essential to note that a global influence on the performance of an organization derives from its managerial culture and the common beliefs and expectations that managers have of the people they oversee [1, 31]. Despite the role they can achieve, it is unavoidable that their influence on the organization can be destructive. Babiak and colleagues [28] concluded that corporate psychopathic were able to get promotions and exert influence in business decision-making in spite of their possibly poor performance. There are "red flags" or "common leadership failures" that may be manifestations of corporate psychopathy. These include disparate treatment of staff, difficulty in forming a team, difficulty in sharing ideas and credit with others [7]. In making an actual overview of the phenomenon, we can say that psychopaths represent about 1% of the general population sample as shown in **Figure 1** [32]; however, Babiak, et al. [28] reported that the prevalence of psychopathy in a sample of high-level managers was about 4%, which is significantly higher than the prevalence found in general samples [32, 33]; other researches even suggest that one in 10 managers are psychopaths (as shown in **Figure 1**) [34, 35]. Some authors [36, 37] have also hypothesized that psychopathy is manifested differently in women than in men, with males displaying more of an "antisocial pattern" and females more of a "histrionic pattern" [35], in any event researchers generally concur that men display higher levels of psychopathy than women do. McWilliams asserts that psychopathy is more common

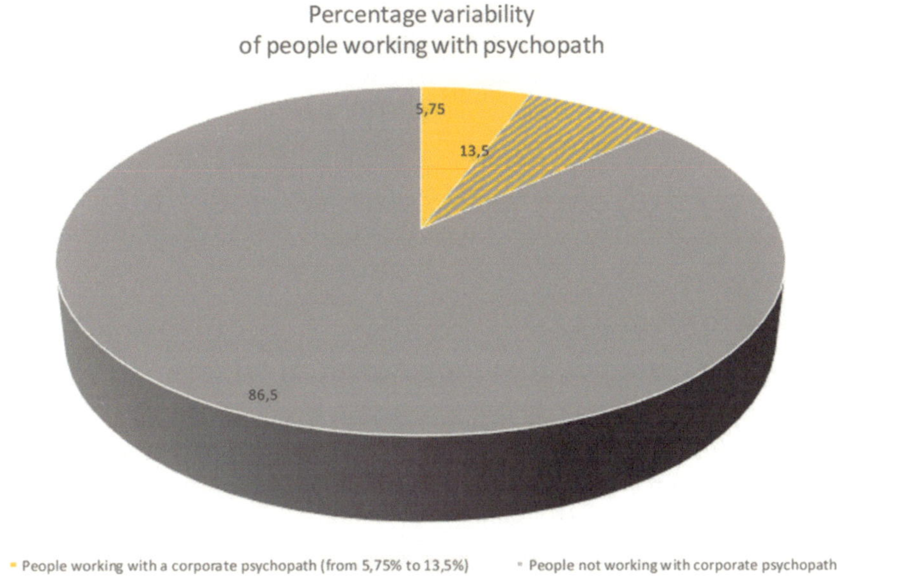

Figure 1. Actual overview of the phenomenon of psychopathy [28, 32, 33].

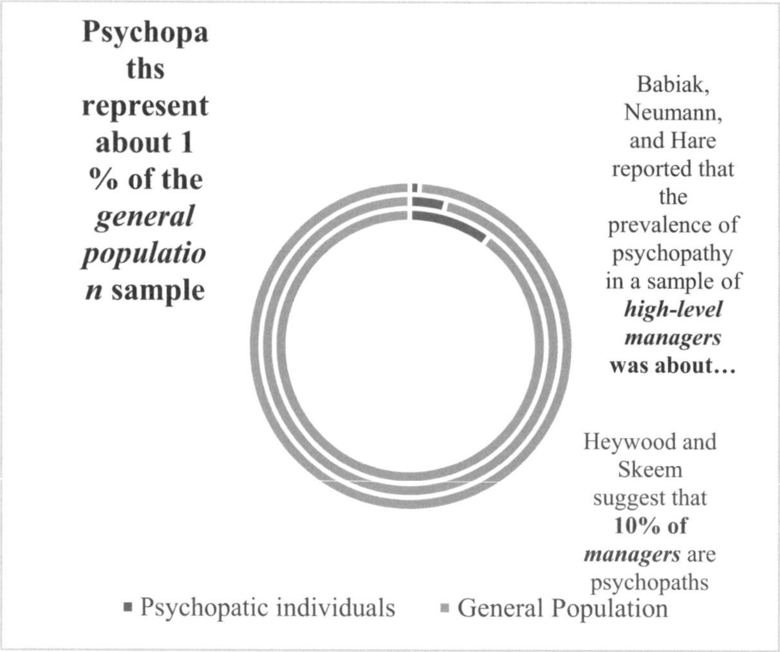

Figure 2. Percentage of employees working with a corporate psychopath [10, 41, 42].

in men probably because females experience realistic limitation earlier (for example they are less physically strong and at greater risk of physical abuse) [23]. Finally we can say that corporate psychopaths are thought to gravitate toward organizations where they can gain money, power, and prestige rather than to the less well-remunerated caring professions [10, 26]: they have been found to be more common in some work categories rather than others, including CEOs and lawyers [10, 38–40]. This level of incidence results in between 5.75 and 13.5% of employees working with a corporate psychopath, as shown in **Figure 2** [10, 41, 42].

Other commentators surprisingly suggest that psychopathy may be beneficial to organizations: these papers and articles should questioned for this viewpoint [10, 25, 43, 44] diverging from the many studies, which we will examine, that verify the importance of preventing these phenomena.

2. General patterns and possible biopsicosocial origins

The variety, number, and intensity of traits differ across persons, hence there can be very significant differences in the behavioral profile of individuals considered to be psychopaths [1]. Independently from the specific traits a general transversal and central dynamic of psychopathic persons is the organizational worry in consciously manipulating or "getting over on" others and the need to exert power that takes precedence over all other aims: the primary defense in psychopathic people is omnipotent control [45, 46]. Psychopathy is generally a clinical construct defined by a cluster of personality traits and characteristics, including shallow emotions, grandiosity, egocentricity, lack of empathy or remorse, deceptiveness, irresponsibility, impulsivity, and a tendency to ignore social norms [47], and thus includes actually a variety of behaviors which reflect violation of societal norms [48]. In the interpersonal domain, the psychopathic person is generally described like grandiose, superficial, and deceitful toward others; in the lifestyle domain, heavy bouts of impulsivity and irresponsibility are frequently reported; in the affective domain this kind of person is conceptualized like without remorse and empathy; and in the antisocial domain, psychopaths generally have a history of exhibiting poor behavioral control and showing antisocial behavior both in adolescence and as an adult [1, 49]. This is a general description but more specifically we can say that there are various psychopathic subtypes that differ for example regarding levels of impulsivity, social cognition, and aggression. Hence they may be more or less successful in society [50, 51], in fact psychopathy is a spectrum rather than a typology, and research using community samples has found individuals to be situated along a "psychopathy continuum" [3, 52]. McWilliams also distinguishes psychopathic thinking to a continuum from psychotic-borderline functioning (defined low level) to a neurotic functioning (defined high level) that is characterized with good-enough ego strength and identity integration, capability to use mature defenses and reality testing [23, 45]: actually variants or subtypes exist, covering a broad range that spans from unsuccessful to very successful. Specifically, corporate psychopaths exhibit subclinical rather than clinical symptoms, with different variations on specific dimensions. Subclinical corporate psychopaths may have some moral emotion deficits, while fully developed psychopaths may instead have more severe moral emotion deficits, and relatively little attachments to others [3], and some senior-ranking managers in "non-criminal" populations have been examined in terms of the construct of "successful psychopathy" [7, 30]; they are said to embody most psychopathic traits, but refrain from serious anti-social behaviors and therefore are infrequently institutionalized [30], in fact although the patterns of dysfunction in their comportment, affect, and cognition are qualitatively the same as conventional conceptualizations of psychopathy, these "subclinical psychopaths" do differ quantitatively in the intensity and pervasiveness of their behavioral disorder [30]. It is not definitively known whether this syndrome derive from physical, biological, or environmental factors [53]; however, patterns of brain dysfunction have been associated with this personality, with particular impairment in the orbital-frontal cortex being evident [54–56], for example, physical damage to some area of the brain can result in the onset of psychopathic behavior and causality is implied but not established [10]. Some authors say instead that sociopathic dynamics are correlated to childhood rife with insecurity and chaos (neglect, harsh discipline, and/or overindulgence) [23, 45]. Exposure to habitual expressions of anger and cruel parenting may provide a model of hostile and aggressive behavior, facilitating the internalization of hostile schemas and access to aggressive responses in both benign and threatening circumstances [57, 58]. Some authors suggest that the exposure of minors to violence and abuse are often risk factors for antisocial behavior in adolescence, as well as the presence of antisocial behavior of parents, which has frequently an adverse impact on the mental health of their children [59]. Research has also suggested that there are some complex interactions between factors, for example some environments can lead to antisocial behavior with low genetic risks (for example profit based societies with high levels of competition and inequality between citizens). Therefore, biological explanations encompassing also psychological events should take into account the complex relationship with belief-systems, cultural values, unique life events, and the social environment, as shown in **Figure 3** [51].

Given its multifactorial origin, and its manifestation influenced by personal variables (such as gender, age, or personality traits) some attempts have been made to clarify some of these specific underlying mechanisms but much work needs to be done to empirically establish clear links [51] and it is important to specify also that the personal biases of investigators will influence their weighing of the potential contributions of the different factors [1]. Finally we note that a perspective that can help to understand this phenomenon, respecting its complexity, is represented by the General Systems Theory, developed by Von Bertalanffy, which considers a set of events interrelated as a system with specific properties and functions depending on the level at which it is located in comparison to a larger system. The systems theory in fact claims that all levels of an organization are interrelated to each other, so that changing one affects the other (as shown in **Figure 3**) [60].

2.1. Specific dynamics in workplace

Individuals considered corporate/organizational/executive psychopaths [1, 2, 7, 61, 62] are also referred to as "snakes in suits" by Babiak and Hare [7], because of their capacity of rising through the ranks to leadership positions, achieving wealth and fame (in some cases) [35]; they have been named "successful" due to their ability to avoid confrontation with legal authorities. In any event, in corporations the term "corporate psychopath" has been adopted as the common term for such people [10, 19, 63, 64]. On the other hand Edwin Sutherland is regarded as the scholar that first (a long time ago) brought the term "white-collar crime" into common usage, describing specific financial crimes committed by some people in the upper socioeconomic position of society [65, 66]. Lykken [67] suggested that there may be some professional

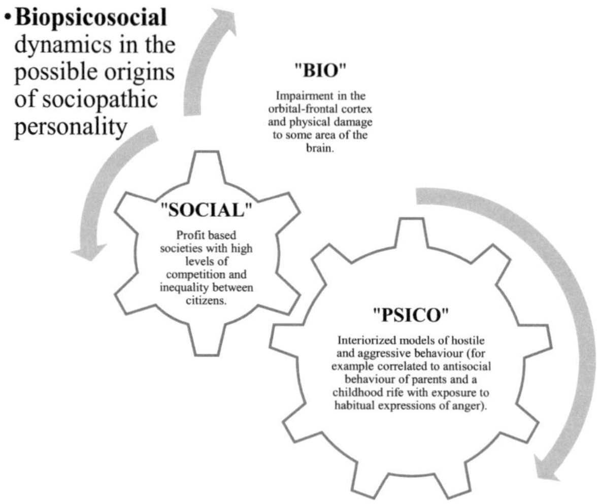

Figure 3. Possible biopsicosocial origins of sociopathic personality [10, 23, 45, 51, 54–60].

advantages to possessing psychopathic inclinations. These professional advantages may be particularly relevant in business, as several of the personality characteristics which speak to the presence of psychopathy are beneficial in finance, including: low anxiety, aggressiveness, self-confidence, charm, dominance, willingness to take risks, and the ability to influence others [7, 68, 69]; in fact through case studies and empirical research, it has been proven that some people with psychopathic traits are capable of excelling in corporate organizations and may be drawn to careers in finance [18, 20, 28, 70, 71]. They may be particularly attracted to the financial power and status gains which are available in senior positions, and can cause considerable damage in such roles by giving course to a manipulative interpersonal style to large-scale fraud [3]: their core ways of acting and thinking show an antisocial sensibility ruthless, even if snakes in suits are apparently well adapted in the higher ranges of organizations, controlling everything and every person in the environment. The concept of corporate psychopathy has been used as a means of understanding unethical behavior in organizations and has often times been associated with bullying, but it is actually quite different from just bullying. Workplace bullying is defined as the repeated unethical and unfavorable treatment of an individual by another in the workplace. This includes behavior aimed ad belittling others through humiliation, threats, sarcasm, overworking a colleague, and rudeness [42, 72, 73]. Bullying can also take the form of applying undue work pressure, sexual harassment and making the victim a "scapegoat" [74]. This behavior is reportedly undertaken to maintain power and control over people [72]. Psychopathic individuals also often brag outright about their power and conquests if they think the listener can be thereby impressed, as a matter of fact one of the most significant characteristic is the possession of a high level of manipulation skills, and the only way they can get other people to understand what they are feeling is to evoke that feeling in them [75, 76]. In the workplace they open appear friendly and pleasant in order to further their goals and provide some measure of emotional reward; they may take pride from having the ability to trick others [1, 7]. Another specific dynamic is the tendency to be high in third-party-directed negative emotions and low in self-directed negative emotions. In other words, they may be frequently giving signals to others to change their behavior but rarely change their own behavior [3]. Other frequent aspects of psychopathic dynamics are: imprudence being this referred to the corporate psychopath's excessive and myopic risk-taking, corruption, capability to conceal risky and often very short-sighted personal agendas which undermine the long term interests of the corporations [77, 78]. However, the corporate psychopath's capacity for concealment also has a crucial weakness: often psychopathic achieve apparent success in their careers, despite negative performance ratings and behaviors potentially harmful to the corporation and its personnel, as a matter of fact some have found psychopathy to be positively related to unethical decision-making: a recurring theme in the business world during the past few years [79, 80].

2.2. Psychosocial aspects and consequences

The workplace can be taken as a model of a complex system, involving psychological, biological and social aspects, so it is necessary to rely on a biopsychosocial approach to deal effectively with any issue concerning individuals and teams. These three dimensions are interlinked, in fact effective management of health and safety in the workplace is important and recommended to individuals and society alike [13], and psychosocial risks should be taken into account when managing the social and environmental contexts that may lead to damages to psychological health [5]. Coherently with these premises, since the end of the 1990s considerable attention and research have been focused on the field of corporate social responsibility worldwide [81]. Psychopathic traits are a potent underlying factor for many of the deviant interpersonal behaviors displayed by some kind of leaders, and a cause of high psychological distress in their colleagues [7]. Bullying in organizations can also lead to a variety of dysfunctional and negative outcomes for the organization as well as for individuals within those organizations [42, 74]: each level of the organization is interconnected with others. Bullying is widespread, inherently unfair to its victims, and is a key ethical problem in modern workplaces [42, 82]. It should also be considered that more often than not there is a link between the actions of toxic managers and its subordinates' deviant conduct [1], on the other hand reciprocal altruism is often beneficial for most of the population because cooperation can increase "survival rates" in the long term even if it reduces opportunities in the short term [3]. While aspects of a psychopathic personality can yield individual success, they may also promote unfavorable emotional reactions in those interacting with psychopaths in the same workplace, resulting in higher psychological distress of other employees [30, 83] and colleagues to be significantly more likely to withdraw in terms of leaving work early and taking longer breaks [10], leading to a decline in global productivity and hence an economic damage to the organization, dynamics that we will deal with. Corporate psychopaths in leadership positions therefore have the potential to adversely influence the lives of many individuals [3] and specifically some psychopathic managers have been assumed to be responsible for their subordinates' reduced job satisfaction, lowered affective engagement, and increased family—work conflict [30, 84, 85]. In addition, Leslie and Van Velsor [86] noted that corporate psychopaths consistently take responsibility for positive outcomes, yet deny responsibility for failure, attributing such results to bad luck or others [30], so they can have a negative impact on employees' moods, psychological well-being, job performances [84], distress [87, 88] and job satisfaction [89, 90]. They prioritize self-interest, which can include destructive consequences such as disruptions to the functioning of a group [3]. Psychopaths have also been described as "homo economicus" [91] because often times they are solely focused on gaining rewards and unconcerned with social consequences; while others may use aggression as an emotional reaction, psychopaths are more likely to use aggression proactively and without emotion: aggressiveness is simply a means to ensure that psychopaths get what they want [3, 92]. These dynamics are counterproductive for the organizations' financial well-being [93], and to be more precise they are associated with a lowering of colleagues' creativity [94], an increase in colleagues' organizational deviance [95] and lowered employee performance [96, 97]. When colleagues are treated unjustly they are more likely to show behaviors that harm the organization or its members [98, 99]. Outcomes also included a marked organizational decline in terms of revenue, employee commitment, inventiveness and organizational innovativeness [10]. Several authors have highlighted a global reduced productivity and increased workplace absenteeism [100]: these deviant workplace behaviors cause losses of billions of dollars across all business organizations, and much of this behavior could possibly stem from corporate psychopaths in positions of leadership [1]; psychopath's behaviors can also affect a company's reputation in the eyes of its customers and employees [6, 7]. In some extreme cases also the surprisingly high number of suicides within organizations could suggest a distorted psychological and managerial environment [1]. We specify also that much of how individuals deal with situations depends on personal coping skills and resources; in fact from the 1960s, there has been a growing awareness on how these aspects make the difference in the outcomes of the adaptation process [101, 102]. The specific features involved in the modulation of the stress-response strategies are called "coping skills," and the whole process of reaction and coping with stress is referred to as "coping" [101, 103]. Prolonged stress situations can be hard tests for such coping skills and it is much more difficult to predict the subjective reactions to them, as well as the possible "burn out." The "burn out" syndrome consists in a dynamic of progressive loss of motivation, idealism, and decreased perception of the social utility of one's own work. The "burn out" condition does not coincide with stress but it induces stress in a work environment when the balance between the following three important factors is lost: (a) required level of performance, (b) control over one's own work, (c) reward and gratification. In some situations, which we just mentioned, it is easier for this balance to be lost [5].

2.3. The importance of prevention: future directions and limits

Based on these findings we underline the importance of primary prevention, the purpose of which is to decrease the incidence of the arisal of the negative phenomenon; primary prevention consists in an attempt to prevent the development of a discomfort in a population at risk [5]. One basic question, which is highly relevant from a practical perspective, is whether there are any instruments that could prevent corporate psychopaths from entering organizations or, when this is not possible, to stop them from climbing the corporate ladder; just because psychopaths are experts at hiding their personality traits, a simple screening procedure during the job interview will probably not detect organizational psychopaths; besides, one has to be experienced and specially trained [53] so it is helpful to build a team of interviewers to tackle hiring procedures; the different perspectives of the team of interviewers can help ensure the decision to be unbiased, and there also should be a sufficient probation period to evaluate performance to prevent any further damage [6, 7]. Specific measures of adult psychopathy are, for example, the Psychopathy Checklist-Revised (PCL-R) [104, 105] and its derivative, the Psychopathy Checklist: Screening Version [106]. For clinical and applied purposes their administration is restricted to those with appropriate professional qualifications (making them unsuitable for use by many human resources personnel). Test administrators need to have high levels of education in psychology or psychology-related fields as well as undergo a comprehensive amount of training given by Hare and his delegates to be considered qualified to administer and interpret results along the appropriate personality dimensions/factors [76]. PCL-R [104, 105], defines psychopathy as a multifaceted construct made up of four dimensions that underpin the superordinate construct of psychopathy [80]: Interpersonal, Affective, Lifestyle, and Antisocial [97]. The proper test typically requires 90–120 minto administer. It consists of different parts: an interview with the subject and a review of the subject's file records and history [49]. It is the person administrating the test who answers a 20-item list. Babiak and Hare developed also the Business-Scan 360 (B-Scan 360). The B-Scan 360 was modeled on a structural model of the PCL-R [104, 105]. In order to make the screening procedure more complete and reach the most straightforward method to offset the limitations inherent in the current standard in detecting psychopathy, a combined approach is recommended, whereby the usage of the tests is complemented with: electroencephalography, measurement of galvanic skin responses, and electromyography [76]. Specifically, it may be useful to observe the correlation between PCL-R scores along with recordings of electroencephalography, galvanic skin responses, and electromyography. To promote secondary and tertiary prevention some authors propose guidelines for how to identify and mitigate the effects of corporate psychopathy [76] already present in the company. The adoption of a program to educate employees in general could be useful [12, 76] for secondary prevention (which tends to reduce the prevalence of morbidity through the curtailment of the period, the spreading of stress) and also tertiary prevention (which tends to mitigate the effects of negative factors on those affected) [5]. It is important to develop proper systems of performance evaluation, based on known criteria (preferably shared), on a transparent communication and on constructive feedback from the management, and also to encourage introspection among employees, so that they can become aware of their own weaknesses (for example predisposition to acquiescence toward stronger personalities) which may be exploited by manipulative corporate psychopaths [76]. The timing of the intervention with the onset of symptoms is, therefore, the discriminating factor between these three levels of prevention [5]. The earlier the preventive intervention takes place, the more effectiveness it has in preventing potential damages. It is also important to discuss the circumstances under which a screening for psychopathy would be morally justified, because only a small percentage of organizational staff will consist of corporate psychopaths: the question is how to avoid a culture of mutual mistrust, where suspicion instead of confidence and collegiality prevails. The suggestion of integrating physiological methods of detection, as well as urging pro-active education of all employees as the symptoms and effects of corporate psychopathy [76] has important practical outcomes, such as identifying job applicants who would be disastrous employees.

3. Conclusions

It is very important to discuss about the specific dynamics, such as manipulation, aggression and cheating behavior, that allow sociopaths to reach leading positions, and on how psychiatry and clinical psychology aim to identify psychopaths in work environments based on these behaviors. The present chapter brings together diverse and growing scientific researches on significant impacts of "business psychopathy" on counterproductive work behavior and ethical decision-making in the corporate world. All the intervention models mentioned could be effective examples of institutional responses to corporate psychopathy dynamics, and this chapter suggests also a framework that may help to identify some risk factors which may be considered in order to safeguard against the potentially damaging behavior of executive psychopaths in organizations. We can also say that the best way to prevent this dynamic is to try the identification before executive psychopaths enter the corporation: once they are established, it will be more difficult to address these dynamics. We specify also that diagnosis is a highly complex issue that needs to be done by mental health professionals. Through appropriate interventions corporations will be able to offer preventive measures with specific educational programs (for example anti-bullying training programs) to promote a certain degree of safety, a team-oriented culture, a culture of prevention and overall increase of the employees' job satisfaction; these preventive measures will promote a degree of immunity to such dangerous dynamics because employees can acquire the tools to identify and deal with executive sociopaths. It is also essential to create a friendly atmosphere of trust for colleagues such that employees can feel comfortable and safe reporting potential behavioral problems. These aspects are particularly important for ethical reasons and also for the economic benefit of corporations: lower employees' turnover and higher employees' job satisfaction will be helpful for productivity and global corporate profit. A boundary that should be noted, and that has already been pointed out by other research [35] is that public policy efforts, such as those directed toward risk assessment, or the pre-employment screening of individuals with marked psychopathic traits, will need to come to grips with the heterogeneity of psychopathy, factor that can make the issue more complicated and difficult to manage. A systematic study of these behaviors will hopefully lead to a higher awareness of society toward the existence of this phenomenon and to a better control of the workplace and social environment.

Author details

Floriana Irtelli[1,2]* and Enrico Vincenti[2,3]

*Address all correspondence to: dott.ssaflorianairtelli@gmail.com

1 Catholic University of the Sacred Heart, Milan, Italy

2 Italian Society of Psychoanalysis of Relation (SIPRe), Italy

3 Department of Psychiatry, Fatebenefratelli Hospital, Cernusco sul Naviglio, Italy

References

[1] Cheang HS, Appelbaum SH. Corporate psychopathy: Deviant workplace behaviour and toxic leaders (part one). Industrial and Commercial Training. 2015;**47**(4):165-173

[2] Boddy CRP. The implications for business performance and corporate social responsibility of corporate psychopaths. American Journal of Behavioral and Brain Science. 2005;**2**(1):30-41

[3] Walker BR, Jackson CJ. Moral emotions and corporate psychopathy: A review. Journal of Business Ethics. 2016;**141**(4):797-810

[4] Stout M. The Sociopath Next Door. New York: Broadway Books; 2005

[5] Ferrari G. Manuale di valutazione dello stress e dei rischi psicosociali [Manual for evaluation of stress and psychosocial risks]. Italy: Edizioni Ferrari Sinibaldi; 2010

[6] Lyon DR, Ogloff JR. Legal and ethical issues in psychopathy assessment. In: Gacono CB, editor. The Clinical and Forensic Assessment of Psychopathy: A Practitioner's Guide. Mahwah, New Jersey: Lawrence Erlbaum Associates Publishers; 2000. p. 139-174

[7] Babiak P, Hare RD. Snakes in Suits: When Psychopaths Go to Work. Chicago: Harper Business; 2006

[8] Strange S. Casino Capitalism. Manchester: Manchester University Press; 1997

[9] McCann L, Morris J, Hassard J. Normalized intensity: The new labour process of middle management. Journal of Management Studies. 2008;**45**(2):343-371

[10] Boddy CRP, Miles D, Sanyal C, Hartog M. Extreme managers, extreme workplaces: Capitalism, organizations and corporate psychopaths. Organization. 2015;**22**(4):530-551

[11] Konrath SH, O'Brien HO, Hsing C. Changes in dispositional empathy in american college students over time: A meta-analysis. Personality and Social Psychology Review. 2010;**20**:1-19

[12] Boddy CRP. The corporate psychopaths theory of the global financial crisis. Journal of Business Ethics. 2011;**102**(2):255-259

[13] EU-OSHA European Agency for Safety and Health at Work [Internet]. 2014. Available from: http://osha.europa.eu; or https://www.healthy-workplaces.eu/en

[14] Cohan WD. This Is how Wall Street Psychopaths Caused the Financial Crisis. [Internet]. 2012. Available from: http://www.businessinsider.com/bill-cohan-an-academic-describes-how-wall-street-psychopaths-caused-thefinancial-crisis-2012-1

[15] Spencer GL, Wargo DT. Malevolent Employees and their Effect on the Ethical Culture of Business Organizations [Internet]. 2010. Available from http://forumonpublicpolicy.com/spring2010.vol2010/spring2010archive/wargo.pdf [Accessed: 2011-12-4]

[16] Ray JJ, Ray JAB. Some apparent advantages of subclinical psychopathy. Journal of Social Psychology. 1982;**117**:135-142

[17] Chiaburu DS, Munoz GJ, Gardner RG. How to spot a careerist early on: Psychopathy and exchange ideology as predictors of careerism. Journal of Business Ethics. 2013;**118**:473-486

[18] Babiak P. When psychopaths go to work: A case study of an industrial psychopath. Applied Psychology. An International Review. 1995;**44**(2):171-188

[19] Babiak P, O'Toole ME. The corporate psychopath. FBI Law Enforcement Bulletin. 2012;**81**(11):7-11

[20] Boddy CRP. The dark side of management decisions: Organisational psychopaths. Management Decision. 2006;**44**(9-10):1461-1475

[21] Morse G. Executive psychopaths. Harvard Business Review. 2004;**82**:20-22

[22] Pech RJ, Slade BW. Organisational sociopaths: Rarely challenged, often promoted. Why? Society and Business Review. 2007;**2**:254-269

[23] McWilliams N. Psychoanalytic Diagnosis, Second Edition: Understanding Personality Structure in the Clinical Process. United States: Guilford Press; 2011

[24] Crawford A. The Pros to Being a Psychopath. [Internet]. 2013. Available from http://www.smithsonianmag.com/science-nature/The-Pros-to-Being-a-Psychopath-176019901.html

[25] Lilienfeld SO, Waldman ID, Landfield K. Fearless dominance and the US presidency: Implications of psychopathic personality traits for successful and unsuccessful political leadership. Journal of Personality and Social Psychology. 2012;(3):489-505

[26] Boddy CRP, Galvin PG, Ladyshewsky R. Leaders without ethics in global business: Corporate psychopaths. Journal of Public Affairs. 2010;**10**(3):121-138

[27] Friedman M. The social responsibility of business is to increase its profits. New York Times. 13 September 1970;32-33

[28] Babiak P, Neumann CS, Hare RD. Corporate psychopathy: Talking the walk. Behavioral Sciences & the Law. 2010;**28**:174-193

[29] Butler JC. The dark triad, employee creativity and performance in new ventures. Frontiers of Entrepreneurship Research. 2015;**35**(3):53-59

[30] Spencer RJ, Byrne MK. Relationship between the extent of psychopathic features among corporate managers and subsequent employee job satisfaction. Personality and Individual Differences. 2016;**101**:440-445

[31] Nica P. Managementul Firmei. Chisinau: Condor Publishing House; 1994

[32] Coid J, Yang M, Ullrich S, Roberts A, Hare RD. Prevalence and correlates of psychopathic traits in the household population of Great Britain. International Journal of Law and Psychiatry. 2009;**32**:65-73

[33] Neumann CS, Hare RD. Psychopathic traits in a large community sample: Links to violence, alcohol use, and intelligence. Journal of Consulting and Clinical Psychology. 2008;**76**:893-899

[34] Heywood L. Corporate Psychopaths. Catalyst (ABC television). Available from: http://www.abc.net.au/catalyst/stories/s1360571.htm. [Accessed: 2005-05-05]

[35] Skeem JL, Polaschek DLL, Patrick CJ, Lilienfeld SO. Psychopathic personality: Bridging the gap between scientific evidence and public policy. Psychological Science in the Public Interest. 2011;**12**(3):95-162

[36] Cloninger CG. The link between hysteria and sociopathy. In: Akiskal SH, Webb W, editors. Psychiatric Diagnosis: Explorations of Biological Predictors. New York, NY: Spectrum; 1978. p. 189-218

[37] Lilienfeld SO, VanValkenberg C, Larntz K, Akiskal HS. The relationship of histrionic personality disorder to antisocial personality disorder and somatization disorders. The American Journal of Psychiatry. 1986;**143**:718-722

[38] Dutton K. Wisdom from psychopaths. Scientific American Magazine. 2013;**23**(6):36-43

[39] Lilienfeld SO, Latzman RD, Watts AL, Smith SF, Dutton K. Correlates of psychopathic personality traits in everyday life: Results from a large community survey. Frontiers in Psychology. 2014;**5**:1-11

[40] Dutton K. The Wisdom of Psychopaths. New York: Random House; 2013

[41] Caponecchia C, Sun A, Wyatt A. Psychopaths' at work? Implications of lay persons' use of labels and behavioural criteria for psychopathy. Journal of Business Ethics. 2011;**107**(4):399-408

[42] Boddy CRP. Corporate psychopaths bullying and unfair supervision in the workplace. Journal of Business Ethics. 2011;**100**:367-379

[43] Smith SF, Watts A, Lilienfeld S. On the trail of the elusive successful psychopath. The Psychologist. 2014;**27**:506-510

[44] Crush P. Every Business Needs a Psychopath. In People Management (CIPD). [Internet]. 2014. Available from: https://the-sps.co.uk/news/news-item/cipd-article-every-business-needs-as-psychopath

[45] McWilliams N. Psychoanalytic Diagnosis: Understanding Personality Structure in the Clinical Process. United States: Guilford Press; 1994

[46] Lingiardi V, Del Corno F, editors. PDM. Manuale diagnostico psicodinamico. Milano: Raffaello Cortina Editore; 2007

[47] Hare RD, Neumann CS. Psychopathy as a clinical and empirical construct. Annual Review of Clinical Psychology. 2008;**4**:217-246

[48] Kazdin A, Buela-Casal G. Conducta Antisocial: Evaluación, Tratamiento y Prevención en la Infancia y Adolescencia [Antisocial Behavior: Evaluation, Treatment and Prevention in Childhood and Adolescence]. Madrid: Pirámide; 1996

[49] Hare RD, Neumann CN. The PCL-R assessment of psychopathy: Development, structural properties, and new directions. In: Patrick C, editor. Handbook of Psychopathy. New York: Guilford; 2006. p. 58-88

[50] Gao Y, Raine A, Schug RA. Event-related potentials and childhood maltreatment in successful and unsuccessful psychopaths. Brain and Cognition. 2011;**77**(2):176-182

[51] Yildirim BO, Derksen JJL. Systematic review, structural analysis, and new theoretical perspectives on the role of serotonin and associated genes in the etiology of psychopathy and sociopathy. Neuroscience and Biobehavioral Reviews. 2013;**37**:1254-1296

[52] Lilienfeld SO, Latzman RD, Watts AL, Smith SF, Dutton K. Correlates of psychopathic personality traits in everyday life: Results from a large community survey. Frontiers in Psychology. 2014;**740**(5):1-11

[53] Hare RD. Predators: The disturbing world of the psychopaths among us. Psychology Today. 1994;**27**(1):54-61

[54] RJR B. Neurocognitive models of aggression, the antisocial personality disorders, and psychopathy. Journal of Neurology, Neurosurgery, and Psychiatry. 2001;**71**(6):727-731

[55] Blair RJR, Cipolotti L. Impaired social response reversal. A case of acquired Sociopathy. Brain. 2000;**123**(6):1122-1141

[56] Perez P. The etiology of psychopathy: A neuropsychological perspective. Aggression and Violent Behavior. 2012;**17**:519-522

[57] Pollak SD, Cicchetti D, Klorman R, Brumaghim JT. Cognitive brain event-related potentials and emotion processing in maltreated children. Child Development. 1997;**68**:773-787

[58] Pollak SD, Cicchetti D, Hornung K, Reed A. Recognizing emotion in faces: Developmental effects of child abuse and neglect. Developmental Psychology. 2000;**36**:679-688

[59] Silberg JL, Maes H, Eaves LJ. Unraveling the effect of genes and environment in the transmission of parental antisocial behavior to children's conduct disturbance, depression and hyperactivity. Journal of Child Psychology and Psychiatry. 2012;**53**:668-677

[60] Engel G. The need for a new medical model: A challenge for biomedicine. Science. 1977;**196**:129-136

[61] Clarke J. The Pocket Psycho. Sydney: Random House; 2007

[62] Newby J. Corporate Psychopaths [Internet]. 2013. Available from: www.abc.net.au/catalyst/stories/s1360571.htm [Accessed: 25 June 2013].

[63] Boddy CRP. A history of research on psychopaths in corporations: The emergence of the corporate psychopath. In: British Academy of Management Annual Conference, British Academy of Management; 13-15 September 2011; Birmingham.

[64] Hare RD. Without Conscience: The Disturbing Word of the Psychopaths among us. 2nd ed. New York: Guilford Press; 1999

[65] Sutherland EH. White Collar Crime. New York: Holt, Rinehart & Winston; 1949

[66] Perri FS. Visionaries or false prophets. Journal of Contemporary Criminal Justice. 2013;**29**(3):331-350

[67] Lykken DT. The Antisocial Personalities. Hillsdale, NJ: Lawrence Erlbaum Associates; 1995

[68] Kernberg O. Regression in organizational leadership. Psychiatry. 1979;**42**:29-39

[69] Yukl G. Leadership in Organisations. Englewood Cliffs, NJ: Prentice Hall; 1981

[70] Henley AG. Psychopathy and career interest in a noncriminal population [Doctoral Dissertation]. Austin: University of Texas; 2001

[71] Wilson MS, McCarthy K. Greed is good? Student disciplinary choice and self-reported psychopathy. Personality and Individual Differences. 2011;**51**(7):873-876

[72] Dierickx C. The bully employee: A survival guide for supervisors. Supervision. 2004; **65**(3):6-7

[73] Djurkovic N, McCormack D, Casimir G. The physical and psychological effects of workplace bullying and their relationship to intention to leave: A test of the psychosomatic and disability hypotheses. International Journal of Organization Theory and Behavior. 2004;**7**(4):469-497

[74] Harvey MG, Buckley MR, Heames JT, Zinko R, Brouer RL, Ferris GR. A bully as an archetypal destructive leader. Journal of Leadership and Organizational Studies. 2007;**14**(2):117-129

[75] Patrick C. Emotion and psychopathy: Startling new insights. Psychophysiology. 2007; **31**(4):319-330

[76] Cheang HS, Appelbaum SH. Corporate psychopathy: Deviant workplace behaviour and toxic leaders (part two). Industrial and Commercial Training. 2015;**47**(5):236-243

[77] Levenson MR, Kiehl KA, Fitzpatrick CM. Assessing psychopathic attributes in a noninstitutionalised population. Journal of Personality and Social Psychology. 1995;**68**:151-158

[78] Schouten R, Silver J. Almost a Psychopath: Do I (or Does Someone I Know) Have a Problem with Manipulation and Lack of Empathy? USA: Harvard University Press; 2012

[79] Stevens GW, Deuling JK, Armenakis AA. Successful psychopaths: Are they unethical decision-makers and why? Journal of Business Ethics. 2012;**105**:139-149

[80] Mathieu C, Hare RD, Jones DN, Babiak P, Neumann CS. Factor structure of the B-scan 360: A measure of corporate psychopathy. Psychological Assessment. 2012;**25**:288-293

[81] Myung JK, Choi YH. The influences of leaders' dark triad trait on their perception of CSR. Asian Journal of Sustainability and Social Responsibility. 2017;1-15

[82] Wornham DA. Descriptive investigation of morality and victimisation at work. Journal of Business Ethics. 2003;**45**(1):29-40

[83] Boddy CRP, Ladyshewsky R, Galvin P. The influence of corporate psychopaths on corporate social responsibility and organisational commitment to employees. Journal of Business Ethics. 2010;**97**:1-19

[84] Spector PE. Job Satisfaction: Application, Assessment, Causes, and Consequences. United States: Thousand Oaks, Sage Publications Inc; 1997

[85] Tepper BJ. Consequences of abusive supervision. Academy of Management Journal. 2000;**43**:178-190

[86] Leslie JB, Van Velsor E. A look at Derailment Today. Greensboro, NC: Center for Creative Leadership; 1996

[87] De Lange AH, Taris TW, Kompier MAJ, Houtman ILD, Bongers PM. The very best of the millennium: Longitudinal research and the demand-control-(support) model. Journal of Occupational Health Psychology. 2003;**8**:282-305

[88] Simon M, Kümmerling A, Hasselhorn HM. Work-home conflict in the European nursing profession. International Journal of Occupational and Environmental Health. 2004;**10**:384-391

[89] Bruck CS, Allen TD, Spector PE. The relation between work–family conflict and job satisfaction: A finer-grained analysis. Journal of Vocational Behavior. 2002;**60**:336-353

[90] Grandey A, Cordeiro B, Crouter A. A longitudinal and multi-source test of the work–family conflict and job satisfaction relationship. Journal of Occupational and Organizational Psychology. 2005;**78**:305-323

[91] Haidt J. The moral emotions. In: Davidson RJ, Scherer KR, Goldsmith HH, editors. Handbook of Affective Sciences. Oxford, UK: Oxford University Press; 2003. p. 852-870

[92] Glenn AL, Raine A. Psychopathy and instrumental aggression: Evolutionary, neurobiological, and legal perspectives. International Journal of Law and Psychiatry. 2009;**32**:253-258

[93] Bensimon H. What to do about anger in the workplace. Training and Development. 1997;**51**:28-32

[94] Liu D, Liao H, Loi R. The dark side of leadership: A three-level investigation of the cascading effect of abusive supervision on employee creativity. Academy of Management Journal. 2012;**55**(5):1187-1212

[95] Tepper BJ, Henle CA, Lambert LS, Giacalone RA, Duffy MK. Abusive supervision and subordinates' organization deviance. The Journal of Applied Psychology. 2008;**93**:721-732

[96] Harris KJ, Kacmar KM, Zivnuska S. An investigation of abusive supervision as a predictor of performance and the meaning of work as a moderator of the relationship. The Leadership Quarterly. 2007;**18**(3):252-263

[97] Mathieu C, Babiak P. Corporate psychopathy and abusive supervision: Their influence on employees' job satisfaction and turnover intentions. Personality and Individual Differences. 2016;**91**:102-106

[98] Aquino K, Galperin BL, Bennett RJ. Social status and interaction between interactional justice and social comparison orientation on antisocial work behaviors aggressiveness as moderators of the relationship between interactional justice and workplace deviance. Journal of Applied Social Psychology. 2004;**34**:1001-1029

[99] Skarlicki DP, Folger R. Retaliation in the workplace: The role of distributive, procedural, and interactional justice. The Journal of Applied Psychology. 1997;**82**:434-443

[100] Clarke J. Working with Monsters: How to Identify and Protect yourself from the Workplace Psychopath. Sydney: Random House; 2005

[101] Lazarus RS, Folkman S. Stress Appraisal and Coping. New York: Springer; 1984

[102] Lazarus RS. Coping theory and research: Past, present and future. Psychosomatic Medicine. 1993;**55**:234-247

[103] Lazarus RS. Psychological Stress and the Coping Process. New York: Mc Graw-Hill; 1966

[104] Hare RD. Manual for the Hare Revised Psychopathy Checklist. 2nd ed. Toronto, Ontario, Canada: Multi-Health Systems; 2003

[105] Neumann CS, Hare RD, Newman JP. The super-ordinate nature of the psychopathy checklist-revised. Journal of Personality Disorders. 2007;**21**:102-117

[106] Hare RD, Neumann CS. Psychopathy and its measurement. In: Corr P, Matthews G, editors. Cambridge Handbook of Personality Psychology. Cambridge: Cambridge University Press; 2009. p. 660-686